KU-647-676

To R.B.W.

Preface

This book is written as a companion to *Respiratory Physiology—The Essentials*, 5th edition (Williams & Wilkins, 1995), and is about the function of the diseased lung as opposed to the normal lung. It is primarily intended for medical students in their second and subsequent years. However, a concise, amply illustrated account of respiratory function in disease may prove useful to the increasingly large number of physicians (anesthesiologists, cardiologists) and paramedical personnel (as well as intensive care personnel and respiratory therapists) who come into contact with respiratory patients. In addition, postgraduate students may find this brief account valuable for reviewing material before examinations.

Many medical schools are constantly trying to emphasize the relevance of the basic science of the first two years to the practice of medicine. Respiratory function can be a model for this. A discussion of a patient with asthma, for example, can quickly and painlessly cover the basic physiology of the airways, blood gases, and lung volumes. It is hoped that this little book will be helpful in such a course that bridges the preclinical and clinical disciplines.

This book emphasizes the relations between structure and function in the diseased lung. Indeed, the reader will find more anatomic pathology than he or she might expect in a book about pathophysiology. However, function cannot be understood properly without a knowledge of structure. It is assumed that students who read this book are also exposed to teaching in pathology.

For this fifth edition, the text has been completely revised and brought up to date in a number of areas, including the pathogenesis of asthma, emphysema, and pulmonary edema. In addition, many sections have been modified, including those on peak expiratory flow rate, closing volume, airway resistance, bronchoactive drugs for the management of asthma, cystic fibrosis, mechanical ventilation, and normal values of pulmonary function tests. However, by judicious pruning, the length of the book has been slightly reduced in sympathy with the plight of modern medical students.

Naturally, such a concise book covering such a wide area must be somewhat dogmatic. However, the reader will find a full discussion of disputed issues in the references and reading list at the end of the book. I would be grateful for any comments on the selection of material and any factual errors.

Contents

Contents

Lung Function Tests and What They Mean

1. Ventilation
2. Gas Exchange
3. Other Tests

We learn how diseased lungs work by doing pulmonary function tests. Accordingly, Part One is devoted to a description of the most important tests and their interpretation. It is assumed that the reader is familiar with the basic physiology of the lung as contained in the companion volume, West JB. Respiratory physiology–the essentials, 5th ed. Baltimore: Williams & Wilkins, 1995.

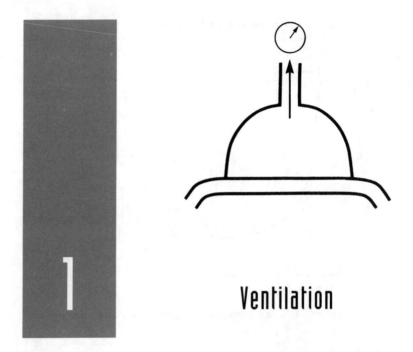

1

Ventilation

The simplest test of lung function is a forced expiration. It is also one of the most informative tests and it requires minimal equipment and trivial calculations. The majority of patients with lung disease have an abnormal forced expiration and, very often, the information obtained from this test is useful in their management. In spite of this, the test is not used as often as it should be. For example, it can be valuable in detecting early airway disease, an extremely common and important condition.

Tests of Ventilatory Capacity

Forced Expiratory Volume

The *forced expiratory volume* (FEV) is the volume of gas exhaled in *one second* by a forced expiration from full inspiration. The *vital capacity* is the *total* volume of gas that can be exhaled after a full inspiration.

A simple way of making these measurements is shown in Figure 1.1. The patient is comfortably seated in front of a spirometer having a low resistance. He or she breathes in maximally and then exhales as hard and as far as he or she can. As the spirometer bell moves up, the kymograph pen moves down, thus indicating the expired volume against time.

Figure 1.2A shows a normal tracing. The volume exhaled in 1 second was 4.0 liters and the total volume exhaled was 5.0 liters. These two volumes are therefore the forced expiratory volume in 1 second (FEV_1) and the vital capacity. The vital capacity measured with a forced expiration may be less than that measured with a slower exhalation, so that the term forced vital capacity (FVC)

Figure 1.1. Measurement of forced expiratory volume (FEV₁) and vital capacity (FVC).

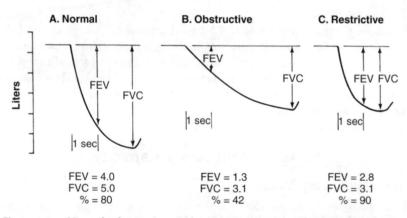

Figure 1.2. Normal, obstructive, and restrictive patterns of a forced expiration.

is generally used. Note that the normal ratio of FEV_1 to FVC is approximately 80%. (See Appendix A for normal values.)

The FEV can be measured over other times, such as 2 or 3 seconds, but the 1-second value is most informative. When the subscript is omitted, the period is 1 second.

Figure 1.2B shows the type of tracing obtained from a patient with chronic obstructive pulmonary disease. Note that the rate at which the air was exhaled was much slower, so that only 1.3 liters were blown out in the first second. In

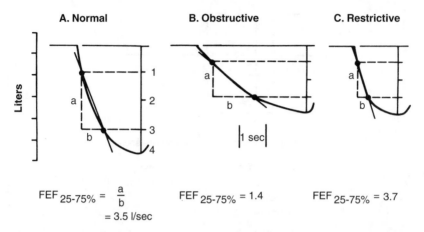

Figure 1.3. Calculation of forced expiratory flow (FEF$_{25-75\%}$) from a forced expiration.

addition, the total volume exhaled was only 3.1 liters. FEV$_1$/FVC was reduced to 42%. These figures are typical of an *obstructive* pattern.

Contrast this pattern with that of Figure 1.2C, which shows the type of tracing obtained from a patient with pulmonary fibrosis. Here the vital capacity was reduced to 3.1 liters, but a large percentage (90%) was exhaled in the first second. These figures mean *restrictive* disease.

The simple water-filled spirometer shown in Figure 1.1 is now seldom used and has been replaced by electronic spirometers, which should provide a graph to be filed with the patient's chart. Careful calibration is important and criteria have been published (1).

The patient should loosen any tight clothing, and the mouthpiece should be at a convenient height. One accepted procedure is to allow two practice blows and then record three good test breaths. The highest FEV$_1$ and FVC from these three breaths are then used. The volumes should be converted to body temperature and pressure (see Appendix A). Further practical details can be found elsewhere (1).

The test is often valuable in assessing the efficacy of bronchodilator drugs. If reversible airway obstruction is suspected, the test should be carried out before and after administering the drug (for example, 0.5% albuterol by nebulizer for 3 minutes). Both the FEV$_1$ and FVC usually increase in a patient with bronchospasm.

Forced Expiratory Flow (FEF$_{25-75\%}$)

This index is calculated from a forced expiration as shown in Figure 1.3. The middle half (by volume) of the total expiration is marked and its duration is measured. The FEF$_{25-75\%}$ is the volume in liters divided by the time in seconds (1).

The correlation between FEF$_{25-75\%}$ and FEV$_1$ is generally close in patients with obstructive pulmonary disease. The changes in FEF$_{25-75\%}$ are often more striking, but the range of normal values is greater.

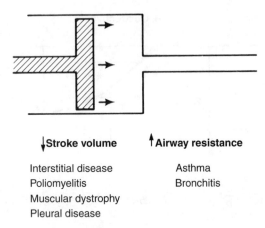

↓Stroke volume	↑Airway resistance
Interstitial disease	Asthma
Poliomyelitis	Bronchitis
Muscular dystrophy	
Pleural disease	

Figure 1.4. Simple model of factors that may reduce the ventilatory capacity. The stroke volume may be reduced by diseases of the lung parenchyma, pleura, or respiratory muscles. Airway resistance is increased in asthma and bronchitis.

Interpretation of Tests of Forced Expiration

In some respects, the lungs and thorax can be regarded as a simple air pump (Fig. 1.4). The output of such a pump depends on the stroke volume, the resistance of the airways, and the force applied to the piston. The last factor is relatively unimportant in a forced expiration, as we shall presently see.

The *vital capacity* (or forced vital capacity) is a measure of the stroke volume, and any reduction in it affects the ventilatory capacity. Causes of stroke volume reduction include diseases of the thoracic cage, such as kyphoscoliosis, ankylosing spondylitis, and acute injuries; diseases affecting the nerve supply to the respiratory muscles or the muscles themselves, such as poliomyelitis or muscular dystrophy; abnormalities of the pleural cavity, such as pneumothorax or pleural thickening; pathology in the lung itself, such as fibrosis, which reduces its distensibility; space-occupying lesions, such as cysts; or an increased pulmonary blood volume, as in left heart failure. In addition, there are diseases of the airways that cause them to close prematurely during expiration, thus limiting the volume that can be exhaled. This occurs in asthma and bronchitis.

The *forced expiratory volume* (and related indices such as the $FEF_{25-75\%}$) is affected by the airway resistance during forced expiration. Any increase in resistance reduces the ventilatory capacity. Causes include bronchoconstriction as in asthma or following the inhalation of irritants, such as cigarette smoke; structural changes in the airways, as in chronic bronchitis; obstructions within the airways, such as an inhaled foreign body or excess bronchial secretions; and destructive processes in the lung parenchyma, which interfere with the radial traction that normally supports the airways.

While the simple model of Figure 1.4 serves as an introduction to the factors limiting the ventilatory capacity of the diseased lung, we need to refine the

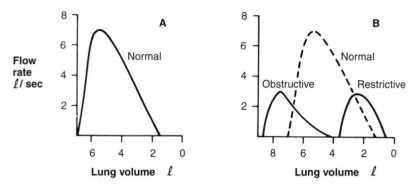

Figure 1.5. **Expiratory flow-volume curves.** (A) Normal. (B) Obstructive and restrictive patterns.

model to obtain a better understanding. For example, the airways are actually *inside* the pump, not *outside*, as shown in Figure 1.4. Useful additional information comes from the flow-volume curve.

Expiratory Flow-Volume Curve

If we record flow rate and volume during a maximal forced expiration, we obtain a pattern like that shown in Figure 1.5A. A curious feature of the flow-volume curve is that it is virtually impossible to get outside it. For example, if we begin by exhaling slowly and then exert maximum effort, the flow rate increases to the envelope but not beyond. Clearly, something very powerful is limiting the maximum flow rate at a given volume. This factor is *dynamic compression of the airways*.

Figure 1.5B shows typical patterns found in obstructive and restrictive lung disease. In obstructive diseases, such as chronic bronchitis and emphysema, the maximal expiration typically begins and ends at abnormally high lung volumes, and the flow rates are much lower than normal. In addition, the curve may have a scooped-out appearance. By contrast, patients with restrictive disease, such as interstitial fibrosis, operate at low lung volumes. Their flow envelope is flattened compared with normal, but if flow rate is related to lung volume, the flow is seen to be higher than normal (Figure 1.5B). Note that the figure shows absolute lung volumes, although these cannot be obtained from a forced expiration. They require an additional measurement of residual volume.

To understand these patterns, consider the pressures inside and outside the airways (Fig. 1.6) (See West JB. Respiratory physiology–the essentials, ed. 5. Baltimore: Williams & Wilkins, 1995: p. 110). Before inspiration (A), the pressures in the mouth, airways, and alveoli are all atmospheric because there is no flow. Intrapleural pressure is, say, 5 cm H_2O below atmospheric pressure, and we assume that the same pressure exists outside the airways (although this is an oversimplification). Thus, the pressure difference expanding the airways is 5 cm H_2O. At the beginning of inspiration (B), all pressures fall and the pressure

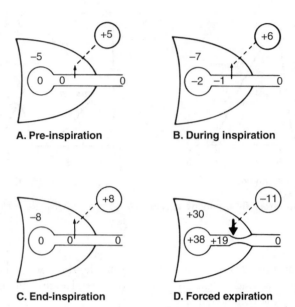

A. Pre-inspiration   B. During inspiration

C. End-inspiration   D. Forced expiration

Figure 1.6. Diagram explaining dynamic compression of the airways during a forced expiration. (See text for details.)

difference holding the airways open increases to 6 cm H_2O. At the end of inspiration (C), this pressure is 8 cm H_2O.

Early in a forced expiration (D), both intrapleural and alveolar pressures rise greatly. The pressure at some point in the airways increases, but not as much as alveolar pressure because of the pressure drop caused by flow. Under these circumstances, we have a pressure difference of 11 cm H_2O tending to *close* the airways. Airway compression occurs, and now flow is determined by the difference between alveolar pressure and the pressure outside the airways at the collapse point (Starling resistor effect). Note that this pressure difference (8 cm H_2O in D) is the static recoil pressure of the lung and is dependent only on lung volume and compliance. It is *independent* of expiratory effort.

How then can we explain the abnormal patterns in Figure 1.5B? In the patient with chronic bronchitis and emphysema, the low flow rate in relation to lung volume is caused by several factors. There may be thickening of the walls of the airways and excessive secretions in the lumen because of bronchitis; both increase the flow resistance. The number of small airways may be reduced because of destruction of lung tissue. Also, the patient may have a reduced static recoil pressure (even though lung volume is greatly increased) because of breakdown of elastic alveolar walls. Finally, the normal support offered to the airways by the traction of the surrounding parenchyma is probably impaired because of loss of alveolar walls, and the airways therefore collapse more easily than they should. These factors are considered in more detail in Chapter 4.

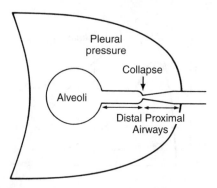

Figure 1.7. Dynamic compression of the airways. When this occurs during a forced expiration, only the resistance of the airways distal to the point of collapse (upstream segment) determines the flow rate. In the last stages of a forced vital capacity, only the peripheral small airways are distal to the collapsed point and therefore determine the flow.

The patient with interstitial fibrosis has normal (or high) flow rates in relation to lung volume because the lung static recoil pressures are high and the caliber of the airways may be normal (or even increased) at a given lung volume. However, because of the greatly reduced compliance of the lung, volumes are very small, and absolute flow rates are therefore reduced.

This analysis shows that Figure 1.4 is a considerable oversimplification and that the forced expiratory volume, which seems so straightforward at first, is affected both by the airways and by the lung parenchyma. Thus, the terms "obstructive" and "restrictive" conceal a good deal of pathophysiology.

Partitioning of Flow Resistance from the Flow-Volume Curve

When the airways collapse during a forced expiration, the flow rate is determined by the resistance of the airways up to the point of collapse (Fig. 1.7). Beyond this point, the resistance of the airways is immaterial. Collapse occurs at (or near) the point where the pressure inside the airways is equal to the intrapleural pressure (*equal pressure point*). This is believed to be in the vicinity of the lobar bronchi early in a forced expiration. However, as lung volume reduces and the airways narrow, their resistance increases. As a result, pressure is lost more rapidly and the collapse point moves into more distal airways. Thus, late in forced expiration, flow is increasingly determined by the properties of the small peripheral airways.

These peripheral airways (say less than 2 mm in diameter) normally contribute less than 20% of the total airway resistance. Therefore, changes in them are difficult to detect and they constitute a "silent zone." However, it is likely that some of the earliest changes in chronic obstructive pulmonary disease occur in these small airways, and therefore maximum flow rate late in a forced expiration is often taken to reflect peripheral airway resistance.

Figure 1.8.   Example of an expiratory flow-volume curve in chronic obstructive pulmonary disease.   Note the scooped-out appearance. The *arrows* show the maximum expiratory flow after 50% and 75% of the vital capacity have been exhaled.

Maximum Flows from the Flow-Volume Curve

Maximum flow ($\dot{V}$max) is frequently measured after 50% ($\dot{V}$max$_{50\%}$) or 75% ($\dot{V}$max$_{75\%}$) of the vital capacity has been exhaled. Figure 1.8 shows an example of the abnormal pattern typically seen in chronic obstructive pulmonary disease. The later in expiration that the flow is measured, the more the measurement reflects the resistance of the very small airways. Some studies have shown abnormalities in the $\dot{V}$max$_{75\%}$ when other indices of a forced expiration, such as the FEV_1 or $FEF_{25-75\%}$, were normal.

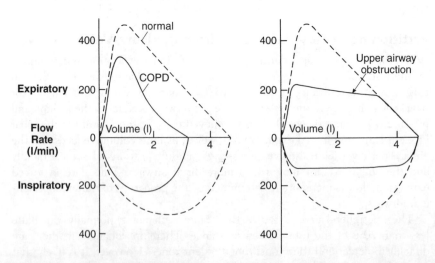

Figure 1.9.   Expiratory and inspiratory flow-volume curves. In normal subjects and patients with chronic obstructive pulmonary disease, inspiratory flow rates are normal (or nearly so). In fixed upper airway obstruction, both inspiratory and expiratory flow rates are reduced.

Peak Expiratory Flow Rate (PEFR)

PEFR is the maximum flow rate during a forced expiration starting from total lung capacity. It can be conveniently estimated with an inexpensive, portable peak flow meter. The measurement is not precise, and it depends on the patient's effort. Nevertheless, it is a valuable tool for following disease, especially asthma, and the patient can easily make repeated measurements in the home or workplace and keep a log to show to the physician.

Inspiratory Flow-Volume Curve

The flow-volume curve is also often measured during inspiration. This curve is not affected by the dynamic compression of the airways because the pressures during inspiration always expand the bronchi (Fig. 1.6). However, the curve is useful in detecting upper airway obstruction, which flattens the curve because maximum flow is limited (Fig. 1.9). Causes include glottic or tracheal stenosis and tracheal narrowing as a result of a compressing neoplasm. The expiratory flow-volume curve is also flattened by fixed (nonvariable) upper airway obstruction.

Airway and Parenchymal Components of the Flow-Volume Curve

We have seen that the forced expiratory volume may be reduced by an increase in airway resistance or a reduced elastic recoil pressure because of parenchymal disease. Is there any way to distinguish between these two factors? One way is to plot the maximum flow rate against the elastic recoil pressure as shown in Figure 1.10. This cannot be done from a forced expiration alone because we

Figure 1.10. Interpretation of a reduced maximum expiratory flow rate. If this is caused solely by parenchymal disease, the normal relationship between maximum flow and recoil pressure is retained. However, increased airway resistance disturbs the relationship.

also need to record esophageal pressure (as a measure of intrapleural pressure) under static conditions at the various lung volumes of the vital capacity. However, the method is described here because it throws light on the interpretation of the flow-volume curve.

If the airways are normal and the reduced flow rate is caused solely by parenchymal disease, the relationship between flow and elastic recoil pressure is unchanged. This pattern is seen (very nearly) in patients thought to have emphysema without bronchitis. However, if the airways are diseased but the parenchyma is normal, the curve departs from the normal range. This pattern is seen in patients with bronchial asthma (Fig. 4.9).

Tests of Uneven Ventilation

Single Breath Nitrogen Test

The tests described so far measure ventilatory capacity. The single breath nitrogen test measures inequality of ventilation. This topic is somewhat different, but is conveniently described here.

Suppose a patient takes a single vital capacity inspiration of oxygen and then exhales slowly to residual volume. If we measure the nitrogen concentration at the mouthpiece with a rapid nitrogen analyzer, we record a pattern as shown in Figure 1.11. Four phases can be recognized. In the first, which is very short, pure oxygen is exhaled from the upper airways and the nitrogen concentration is zero. In the second phase, nitrogen concentration rises rapidly as the anatomic dead space is washed out by alveolar gas. This phase is also short.

The third phase consists of alveolar gas, and the tracing is almost flat in normal subjects. This portion is often known as the alveolar plateau. In patients with uneven ventilation, the third phase steadily rises, and the slope is a measure of the inequality of ventilation. It is expressed as the percentage increase in nitrogen concentration per liter of expired volume; the range of normal values is given in Appendix A. In carrying out this test, the expiratory flow rate should be less than 0.5 liters/sec in order to reduce the variability of the results.

The reasons for the rise in nitrogen concentration in phase 3 are not fully understood. Apparently, some regions of lung are ventilated poorly and therefore receive relatively little of the breath of oxygen. These areas therefore have a relatively high concentration of nitrogen because there is less oxygen to dilute this gas. Also, these poorly ventilated regions tend to empty last.

Three possible mechanisms are shown in Figure 1.12. In A, the region is poorly ventilated because of partial obstruction of its airway and, because of this high resistance, the region empties late. In fact, the rate of emptying of such a region is determined by its time constant, which is given by the product of its airway resistance (R) and compliance (C). The larger the time constant (RC), the longer it takes to empty. This mechanism is known as *parallel* inequality of ventilation.

Figure 1.12B shows a different mechanism known as *series* inequality. Here there is a dilation of peripheral airspaces causing differences of ventilation *along*

Figure I.II. Single breath nitrogen test of uneven ventilation. Note the four phases of the expired tracing. *CV*, closing volume. (See text for details.)

Figure I.12. Three mechanisms of uneven ventilation. In parallel inequality *(A)*, flow to regions with long time constants is reduced. In series inequality *(B)*, dilation of a small airway may result in impaired diffusion along a terminal lung unit. Collateral ventilation *(C)* may also cause series inequality.

the air passages of a lung unit. In this context, we should recall that inspired gas reaches the terminal bronchioles by convective flow, that is, like water running through a hose, but its subsequent movement to the alveoli is chiefly accomplished by diffusion within the airways. Normally, the distances are so short that nearly complete equilibration of gas concentrations is established quickly. However, if the small airways enlarge, as occurs, for example, in centriacinar emphysema (Fig. 4.4), the concentration of inspired gas in the most distal airways remains low. Again, these poorly ventilated regions empty last.

Figure 1.12C shows another form of series inequality that occurs when some lung units receive their inspired gas from neighboring units rather than from the large airways. This is known as collateral ventilation and appears to be an important process in chronic obstructive pulmonary disease.

There is still uncertainty about the relative importance of parallel and series inequality. It is likely that both operate to some extent in normal subjects and in a much exaggerated form in patients with obstructive pulmonary disease. Whatever the mechanism, the single breath nitrogen test is a simple, rapid, and reliable way of measuring the degree of uneven ventilation in the lung. This is increased in most obstructive and many restrictive types of lung disease (see Chapters 4 and 5).

Closing Volume

Toward the end of the vital capacity expiration shown in Figure 1.11, the nitrogen concentration rises abruptly, signaling the onset of airway closure, or phase 4. The lung volume at which phase 4 begins is called the *closing volume*, and the closing volume plus the residual volume is known as the *closing capacity*. In practice, the onset of phase 4 is obtained by drawing a straight line through the alveolar plateau (phase 3) and noting the last point of departure of the nitrogen tracing from this line.

Unfortunately, the junction between phases 3 and 4 is seldom as clear-cut as in Figure 1.11, and there is considerable variation of this volume when repeated measurements are made on the same patient. The test is most useful in the presence of small amounts of disease because severe disease distorts the tracing so much that the closing volume cannot be identified.

The mechanism of the onset of phase 4 is still uncertain, but many people believe that it is caused by closure of small airways in the lowest part of the lung. At residual volume just before the single breath of oxygen, the nitrogen concentration is virtually uniform throughout the lung, but the basal alveoli are much smaller than the apical alveoli in the upright subject because of distortion of the lung by its weight. Indeed, the lowest portions are compressed so much that the small airways in the region of the respiratory bronchioles are closed. However, at the end of a vital capacity inspiration, all the alveoli are approximately the same size. Thus, the nitrogen at the base is diluted much more than that of the apex by the breath of oxygen.

During the subsequent expiration, the upper and lower zones empty together and the expired nitrogen concentration is nearly constant (Fig. 1.11). As soon as dependent airways begin to close, however, the higher nitrogen concentration in the upper zones preferentially affects the expired concentration, causing an abrupt rise. Moreover, as airway closure proceeds up the lung, the expired nitrogen progressively increases.

Recent studies show that in some subjects, the closing volume is the same in the weightlessness of space as in normal gravity (2). This finding suggests that compression of dependent lung is not the mechanism, and it emphasizes how uncertain we are about this topic.

The volume at which airways close is very age-dependent, being as low as 10% of the vital capacity in young normal subjects but increasing to 40%, (i.e., approximately the FRC) at about the age of 65 years. There is some evidence that the test is sensitive to small amounts of disease. For example, apparently healthy cigarette smokers sometimes have increased closing volumes when their ventilatory capacity is normal.

Other Tests of Uneven Ventilation

Uneven ventilation can also be measured by a multibreath nitrogen washout during oxygen breathing. Topographic inequality of ventilation can be determined using radioactive xenon. The present chapter is confined to single breath tests; these other measurements are covered in Chapter 3.

Tests of Early Airway Disease

There has been great interest in the possible use of some of the tests described in this chapter to identify patients with early airway disease. Once a patient develops the full picture of chronic obstructive pulmonary disease, the results of treatment are generally disappointing. The hope is that by identifying disease at an early stage, its progression can be slowed, for example, by the patient stopping cigarette smoking.

Among the tests that have been examined in this context are the FEV_1, $FEF_{25-75\%}$, $\dot{V}max_{50\%}$ and $\dot{V}max_{75\%}$, and the closing volume. Assessment of these tests is difficult because it depends on prospective studies and large control groups. Although work continues, it is clear that the original test of FEV_1 remains one of the most reliable and valuable tests. While more sophisticated tests should clearly be investigated, measuring the FEV_1 and FVC remains mandatory.

2

Gas Exchange

Chapter 1 dealt with the simplest test of lung function: the forced expiration. In addition, we looked briefly at other single breath tests of uneven ventilation. In this chapter, we turn to the most important measurement in the management of respiratory failure: arterial blood gases. Another test of gas exchange, the diffusing capacity, is also discussed.

Blood Gases

Arterial Po$_2$

Measurement

It is often essential to know the partial pressure of oxygen in the arterial blood of acutely ill patients. With modern blood gas electrodes, the measurement of arterial Po$_2$ is relatively simple, and the test should be available in all hospitals where patients with respiratory failure are managed.

Arterial blood is usually taken by puncture of the radial artery or from an indwelling radial artery catheter. The dead space of the syringe should be filled with dilute heparin, and ideally the blood should be analyzed within a few minutes. If this is not possible, the syringe should be placed in a beaker of ice to slow down the metabolism of the blood.

Figure 2.1.   Oxygen and carbon dioxide electrodes. In both instances, the blood sample is separated from the electrode by a semipermeable membrane. The electrodes are connected to an amplifier, which reads out the P_{O_2} and P_{CO_2} directly. (Modified from Cotes JE. Lung Function. 5th ed. Oxford: Blackwell, 1993.)

Arterial P_{O_2} is measured with a polarographic oxygen electrode (Fig. 2.1). The principle is that if a small voltage (0.6 volt) is applied to a platinum electrode immersed in a buffer solution, the current that flows is proportional to the P_{O_2}. In practice, the buffer is separated from the blood by a semipermeable membrane through which oxygen diffuses. Oxygen is consumed by the electrode; consequently, the measured P_{O_2} falls with time. The fall is fastest when the P_{O_2} is high. The electrode is calibrated with gas or with a solution of known P_{O_2} (3).

Normal Values

The normal value for P_{O_2} in young adults averages approximately 95 mm Hg, with a range of approximately 85–100. The normal value falls steadily with age, and the average is approximately 85 mm Hg at age 60 years (see Appendix A). The cause of the fall in P_{O_2} with age is probably increasing ventilation–perfusion inequality (see below).

Whenever we read a report of an arterial P_{O_2}, we should have the oxygen dissociation curve at the back of our mind. Figure 2.2 reminds us of two anchor points on the normal curve–arterial blood (P_{O_2} 100, O_2 saturation 97%) and mixed venous blood (P_{O_2} 40, O_2 saturation 75%). Also, we should recall that above 60 mm Hg, the curve is fairly flat and cyanosis is probably undetectable. The curve is shifted to the right by an increase in temperature and P_{CO_2} and a fall in pH (these all occur in exercising muscle where enhanced unloading of O_2 is advantageous). The curve is also shifted to the right by an increase in 2,3-diphosphoglycerate (DPG) inside the red cells. 2,3 DPG is depleted in stored blood but is increased in prolonged hypoxia.

Figure 2.2. Anchor points of the oxygen dissociation curve. The curve is shifted to the right by an increase in temperature, P_{CO_2}, 2,3-DPG, and a fall in pH. The oxygen concentration scale is based on a hemoglobin concentration of 14.5 g/100 ml.

Causes of Hypoxemia

There are four primary causes of a reduced P_{O_2} in arterial blood:

1. Hypoventilation
2. Diffusion impairment
3. Shunt
4. Ventilation–perfusion inequality

A fifth cause, reduction of inspired P_{O_2}, such as during residence at high altitude or breathing a mixture of low oxygen concentration, is seen only in special circumstances.

Hypoventilation

This means that the volume of fresh gas going to the alveoli per unit time (alveolar ventilation) is reduced. If the resting oxygen consumption is not correspondingly reduced, hypoxemia inevitably results. Hypoventilation is commonly caused by diseases outside the lungs; indeed, very often the lungs are normal.

Two cardinal physiologic features of hypoventilation should be emphasized. First, it *always* causes a rise in P_{CO_2} and this is a valuable diagnostic feature. The relationship between the arterial P_{CO_2} and the level of alveolar ventilation in the normal lung is a simple one:

$$P_{CO_2} = \frac{\dot{V}_{CO_2}}{\dot{V}_A} \cdot K \qquad \text{(Eq. 2.1)}$$

where $\dot{V}_{CO_2}$ is the CO_2 output, $\dot{V}_A$ is the alveolar ventilation, and K is a constant (see Appendix A for a list of symbols). This means that if the alveolar ventilation is halved, the P_{CO_2} is doubled. If the patient does not have a raised arterial P_{CO_2}, he or she is not hypoventilating!

Second, the hypoxemia can be abolished easily by increasing the inspired P_{O_2} by delivering oxygen via a face mask. This can be seen from the *alveolar gas equation*:

$$P_{A_{O_2}} = P_{I_{O_2}} - \frac{P_{A_{CO_2}}}{R} + F \qquad \text{(Eq. 2.2)}$$

where F is a small correction factor that we shall ignore. This equation states that if the arterial P_{CO_2} (P_{aCO_2}) and respiratory exchange ratio (R) remain constant (they will if the alveolar ventilation and metabolic rate remain unaltered), every mm Hg rise in inspired P_{O_2} ($P_{I_{O_2}}$) produces a corresponding rise in alveolar P_{O_2} ($P_{A_{O_2}}$). Because it is easily possible to increase the inspired P_{O_2} by several hundred mm Hg, the hypoxemia of pure hypoventilation can readily be abolished.

It is also important to appreciate that the arterial P_{O_2} cannot fall to very low levels from pure hypoventilation. Referring to Equation 2.2 again, we can see that if R = 1, the alveolar P_{O_2} falls 1 mm Hg for every 1 mm Hg rise in P_{CO_2}. This means that severe hypoventilation sufficient to double the P_{CO_2} from 40 to 80 mm Hg only decreases the alveolar P_{O_2} from, say, 100 to 60 mm Hg. If R = 0.8, the fall is somewhat greater, say, to 50 mm Hg. Also, the arterial P_{O_2} is usually a few mm Hg lower than the alveolar value. Even so, the arterial O_2 saturation will be near 80% and cyanosis will probably be just detectable (Fig. 2.3). However, this is a severe degree of CO_2 retention, which may result in substantial respiratory acidosis, with a pH of around 7.2 and a very sick patient! Thus, hypoxemia is not the dominant feature of hypoventilation.

The causes of hypoventilation are shown in Figure 2.4. They include: 1) depression of the respiratory center by drugs (especially barbiturate and morphine derivatives) or anesthesia; 2) diseases of the medulla including encephalitis, trauma, hemorrhage, or neoplasm (rare); 3) abnormalities of the spinal conducting pathways, as following high cervical dislocation; 4) anterior horn cell diseases, such as poliomyelitis; 5) diseases of the nerves to the respiratory muscles, including the Guillain-Barré syndrome and diphtheria; 6) diseases of the myoneural junction, such as myasthenia gravis and anticholinesterase poisoning; 7) diseases of the respiratory muscles, for example, progressive muscular dystrophy; 8) thoracic cage abnormalities, such as crushed chest; and 9) upper airway obstruction, such as tracheal compression by a thymoma.

In addition, hypoventilation is seen in some extremely obese patients who also have somnolence, polycythemia, and excessive appetite. This has been dubbed the "pickwickian syndrome" after the fat boy, Joe, in Charles Dickens' *Pickwick Papers*. The cause of the hypoventilation is uncertain, but the increased

Figure 2.3. Gas exchange during hypoventilation. Values are approximate only.

Figure 2.4. Causes of hypoventilation. (See text for details.)

work of breathing associated with obesity is probably a factor, although some patients appear to have an abnormality of the central nervous system. There is also a rare condition of idiopathic hypoventilation of unknown cause.

Sleep apnea can be divided into *central*, in which there are no respiratory efforts, and *obstructive*, in which, despite activity of the respiratory muscles, there is no airflow.

Central sleep apnea often occurs in patients with hypoventilation because respiratory drive is depressed during sleep. During REM sleep, breathing is often irregular and unresponsive to chemical and vagal drives. An exception is hypoxemia, which usually remains a powerful stimulus to breathe.

Obstructive sleep apnea is much more common than was once thought. The first reports were in extremely obese patients, but it is now recognized that the condition is not confined to them. Airway obstruction can be caused by backward movement of the tongue, collapse of the pharyngeal walls, greatly enlarged tonsils or adenoids, and other anatomic causes of pharyngeal narrowing. Loud snoring often occurs, and the patient may wake violently after an apneic episode. Chronic sleep deprivation sometimes occurs, and the patient may have daytime somnolence, impaired cognitive function, chronic fatigue, morning headaches, and personality disturbances, such as paranoia, hostility, and agitated depression.

A condition affecting infants is the *sudden infant death syndrome* (SIDS). Here the child is typically found dead in the crib with no apparent cause. The etiology of this syndrome is still obscure. One hypothesis is that the nervous control of ventilation is not fully developed and the respiratory muscles are poorly coordinated.

Diffusion Impairment

This means that equilibration does not occur between the P_{O_2} in the pulmonary capillary blood and alveolar gas. Figure 2.5 reminds us of the time course for

Figure 2.5.   Changes in P_{O_2} along the pulmonary capillary. On exercise, the time available for O_2 diffusion across the blood-gas barrier is reduced. A thickened alveolar wall slows the rate of diffusion.

P_{O_2} along a pulmonary capillary. Under normal resting conditions, the capillary blood P_{O_2} almost reaches that of alveolar gas after about 1/3 of the total contact time of 3/4 second available in the capillary. Thus, there is plenty of time in reserve. Even with severe exercise when the contact time may be reduced to as little as 1/4 second, equilibration is virtually assured.

However, in some diseases, the blood-gas barrier is thickened and diffusion is so slowed that equilibration may be incomplete. Figure 2.6 shows a histologic section of lung from a patient with interstitial fibrosis (4). Note that the normally delicate alveolar walls are grossly widened. In such a lung, we expect a slower time course as shown in Figure 2.5. Any hypoxemia that occurred at rest would be exaggerated on exercise because of the reduced contact time.

Diseases in which diffusion impairment may contribute to the hypoxemia, especially on exercise, include asbestosis, sarcoidosis, diffuse interstitial fibrosis including idiopathic pulmonary fibrosis (cryptogenic fibrosing alveolitis) and interstitial pneumonia, connective tissue diseases affecting the lung including scleroderma, rheumatoid lung, lupus erythematosus, Wegener's granulomatosis, Goodpasture's syndrome, and alveolar cell carcinoma. In all these conditions, the diffusion path from alveolar gas to red blood cell may be increased, at least in some regions of the lung, and the time course for oxygenation may be affected, as shown in Figure 2.5.

However, the importance of diffusion impairment to the arterial hypoxemia of these patients is uncertain. As has been emphasized, the normal lung has lots of diffusion time in reserve. In addition, if we look at Figure 2.6, it is impossible to believe that the normal relationships between ventilation and blood flow can be preserved in a lung with such an abnormal architecture. We shall see shortly that ventilation–perfusion inequality is a powerful cause of hypoxemia, which is undoubtedly operating in these patients. Thus, how much additional hypoxemia should be attributed to diffusion impairment is difficult to know. It is clear that at least some of the hypoxemia on exercise is caused by this mechanism (Figure 5.6).

Another possible way in which hypoxemia could result would be an extreme reduction in contact time. Suppose that so much blood flow is diverted away from other regions of the lung (for example, by a large pulmonary embolus) that the time for oxygenation within the capillary is reduced to one-tenth normal. Figure 2.5 shows that hypoxemia would then be inevitable. Whether this ever occurs in practice is unknown.

Any hypoxemia caused by diffusion impairment can be corrected readily by administering 100% oxygen to the patient. The resultant large increase in alveolar P_{O_2} of several hundred mm Hg can easily overcome the increased diffusion resistance of the thickened alveolar membrane. Carbon dioxide elimination is generally thought to be unaffected by diffusion abnormalities, although recent work has raised questions about this subject. Certainly, most patients with the diseases listed previously do not have carbon dioxide retention. Indeed, typically the arterial P_{CO_2} is slightly lower than normal because ventilation is overstimulated, either by the hypoxemia or by intrapulmonary stretch receptors.

Figure 2.6. Section of lung from a patient with diffuse interstitial fibrosis. Note the extreme thickening of the alveolar walls, which constitutes a barrier to diffusion (compare with Figures 5.1, 5.3, and 10.5). (From Hinson KFW. Diffuse pulmonary fibrosis. Hum Pathol 1970;1:275–288.)

Shunt

This means that some blood reaches the arterial system without passing through ventilated regions of the lung. Intrapulmonary shunts can be caused by arterial-venous fistulas, although these are rare. In addition, a completely unventilated but perfused area of lung, for example, a consolidated pneumonic lobule, constitutes a shunt. It might be argued that the latter example is simply one extreme of the spectrum of ventilation–perfusion ratios and that it is therefore more reasonable to classify hypoxemia caused by this under the heading of ventilation–perfusion inequality. However, shunt causes such a characteristic pattern of gas exchange during 100% oxygen breathing that it is convenient to include unventilated alveoli under this heading. Very large shunts are often seen in the adult respiratory distress syndrome (see Chapter 8). Many shunts are extrapulmonary, including those that occur in congenital heart disease through atrial or ventricular septal defects or a patent ductus arteriosus. In such patients, there must be a rise in right heart pressure; otherwise the shunt is from left to right.

If a patient with a shunt is given pure oxygen to breathe, the arterial P_{O_2} fails to rise to the level seen in normal subjects. Figure 2.7 shows that while the end-capillary P_{O_2} may be as high as that in alveolar gas, the O_2 concentration of the shunted blood is as low as in venous blood. When a small amount of shunted blood is added to arterial blood, the O_2 concentration is therefore depressed. This causes a large fall in arterial P_{O_2} because the O_2 dissociation curve is so flat in its upper range. As a result, it is possible to detect small shunts by measuring the arterial P_{O_2} during 100% O_2 breathing.

Only shunts behave in this way, a point of great practical importance. In the other three causes of hypoxemia, hypoventilation, diffusion impairment, and ventilation–perfusion inequality, the arterial P_{O_2} nearly reaches the level seen in normal subjects during 100% O_2 breathing. This may take a long time in some patients who have poorly ventilated alveoli because the nitrogen takes so long to wash out completely that the P_{O_2} is slow to reach its final level. This is

Figure 2.7. Shunt during 100% O₂ breathing. The addition of a small amount of shunted blood with its low O₂ concentration greatly reduces the Po₂ of arterial blood. This is because the O₂ dissociation curve is so flat when the Po₂ is high.

probably the reason why the arterial P_{O_2} of patients with chronic obstructive pulmonary disease may only rise to 400–500 mm Hg after 15 minutes of 100% O_2 breathing.

The magnitude of the shunt during O_2 breathing can be determined from the *shunt equation:*

$$\frac{\dot{Q}s}{\dot{Q}T} = \frac{C'_c - C_a}{C'_c - C_{\bar{v}}} \qquad \text{(Eq. 2.3)}$$

where $\dot{Q}s$ and $\dot{Q}T$ refer to the shunt and total blood flows, and C'_c, C_a and $C_{\bar{v}}$ refer to the O_2 concentrations of end-capillary, arterial, and mixed venous blood. The O_2 concentration of end-capillary blood is calculated from the alveolar P_{O_2} assuming complete equilibration between the alveolar gas and the blood. Mixed venous blood is sampled with a catheter in the pulmonary artery. Alternatively, the denominator in Equation 2.3 can be calculated from the measured oxygen uptake and cardiac output. Sometimes a figure of 5 ml/100 ml is assumed, but this can lead to substantial errors.

Shunt does not usually result in a raised arterial P_{CO_2}. The tendency for this to rise is generally countered by the chemoreceptors which increase ventilation if the P_{CO_2} increases. Indeed, often the arterial P_{CO_2} is lower than normal because of the additional hypoxemic stimulus to ventilation.

Ventilation–perfusion Inequality

This means that ventilation and blood flow are mismatched in various regions of the lung, with the result that all gas transfer becomes inefficient. This mechanism of hypoxemia is extremely common; it is responsible for most, if not all, of the hypoxemia of chronic obstructive pulmonary disease, interstitial lung disease, and vascular disorders such as pulmonary embolism. It is generally identified by excluding the other three causes of hypoxemia: hypoventilation, diffusion impairment, and shunt.

All lungs have some ventilation–perfusion inequality. In the normal upright lung, this takes the form of a regional pattern, with the ventilation–perfusion ratio decreasing from apex to base. But as disease occurs and progresses, we see a disorganization of this pattern until eventually the normal relationships between ventilation and blood flow are destroyed at the alveolar level. (For a discussion of the physiology of how ventilation–perfusion inequality causes hypoxemia, the reader is referred to the companion volume, West JB. Respiratory physiology–the essentials, ed. 5: pp. 57–69.)

Several factors can exaggerate the hypoxemia of ventilation–perfusion inequality. One is concomitant hypoventilation, which may occur, for example, if a patient with severe chronic obstructive pulmonary disease is overly sedated. Another factor that is frequently overlooked is a reduction in cardiac output. This causes a fall of P_{O_2} in mixed venous blood, which results in a fall of arterial P_{O_2} for the same degree of ventilation–perfusion inequality. This situation may be seen in patients who develop a myocardial infarct with mild pulmonary edema.

How can we assess the severity of ventilation–perfusion inequality from the arterial blood gases? First, the *arterial Po₂* is a useful guide. A patient with an arterial P_{O_2} of 40 mm Hg is likely to have more ventilation–perfusion inequality than a patient with an arterial P_{O_2} of 70 mm Hg. However, we can be misled. For example, suppose that the first patient had reduced his or her ventilation, with the result that the alveolar P_{O_2} had fallen by 30 mm Hg, thus pulling down the arterial P_{O_2}. Under these conditions, the arterial P_{O_2} by itself would be deceptive. For this reason, we often calculate the *alveolar–arterial difference* for P_{O_2}.

What should we use for alveolar P_{O_2}? Figure 2.8 reminds us that in a lung with ventilation–perfusion ($\dot{V}_A/\dot{Q}$) inequality, there may be a wide spectrum of values for alveolar P_{O_2} ranging from inspired gas to mixed venous blood. Riley and Cournand (5) suggested that we calculate an "ideal alveolar P_{O_2}." This is the value that the lung *would* have if there were no ventilation–perfusion inequality and if the respiratory exchange ratio remained the same. It is found from the alveolar gas equation:

$$P_{A_{O_2}} = P_{I_{O_2}} - \frac{Pa_{CO_2}}{R} + F \qquad \text{(Eq. 2.4)}$$

using the respiratory exchange ratio R of the whole lung, and assuming that arterial and alveolar P_{CO_2} are the same (usually they nearly are). Thus, the *alveolar-arterial difference* for P_{O_2} makes an allowance for the effect of any under-ventilation or overventilation on the arterial P_{O_2} and is a purer measure of ventilation–perfusion inequality. Other indices include the physiologic dead space and physiologic shunt (See West JB. Respiratory physiology–the essentials, ed. 5: pp. 158–159 for further details.)

It is possible to obtain more information about the distribution of ventilation–perfusion ratios in the lung with a technique based on the elimination of injected

Figure 2.8.   O₂–CO₂ diagram showing the mixed venous (v̄), inspired (I), arterial, ideal, alveolar, and expired points. The *curved line* indicates the Po₂ and Pco₂ of all lung units having different ventilation–perfusion ($\dot{V}_A/\dot{Q}$) ratios. (For additional information on this difficult topic, see West JB. Respiratory physiology, the essentials, ed. 5. Baltimore: Williams & Wilkins, 1995: pp. 157–159.)

foreign gases (6). A series of six inert gases dissolved in saline is slowly infused into a peripheral vein, and after a steady state of elimination by the lung has been achieved, the concentrations are measured in the arterial blood and expired gas by gas chromatography. Because the gases have different solubilities, they partition themselves between blood and gas according to the ventilation–perfusion ratio of the lung unit. It is thus possible to derive a virtually continuous distribution of ventilation–perfusion ratios that is consistent with the measured pattern of elimination of the six gases. Figure 2.9 shows a typical pattern found in young normal volunteers; it can be seen that almost all the ventilation and blood flow go to lung units with ventilation–perfusion ratios near the normal value of 1. As we shall see subsequently, this pattern is greatly disturbed by lung disease.

Mixed Causes of Hypoxemia

These frequently occur. For example, a patient who is being mechanically venti-lated because of acute respiratory failure after an automobile accident may have a large shunt through unventilated lung in addition to severe ventilation–perfusion inequality (Fig. 8.3). Again, a patient with interstitial lung disease may have some diffusion impairment, but this is certainly accompanied by ventilation–perfusion inequality and possibly by shunt as well (Figure 5.6). In our present state of knowledge, it is often impossible to define accurately the mechanism of hyp-oxemia, especially in the acutely ill patient.

Figure 2.9.   Example of a distribution of ventilation–perfusion ratios in a young normal subject as obtained by the multiple inert gas elimination technique. Note that most of the ventilation and blood flow go to lung units with ventilation–perfusion ratios near 1. (From Wagner PD, Laravuso RB, Uhl RR, West JB. Continuous distributions of ventilation–perfusion ratios in normal subjects breathing air and 100% O_2. J Clin Invest 1974;54:54–68.)

Oxygen Delivery to Tissues

Although the P_{O_2} of arterial blood is of great importance, other factors enter into the delivery of oxygen to the tissues. For example, a reduced arterial P_{O_2} in a patient with a hemoglobin of 5g/100 ml is clearly more detrimental than in a patient with a normal O_2 capacity. The delivery of oxygen to the tissues depends on the oxygen capacity of the blood, the cardiac output, and the distribution of blood flow to the periphery. These factors are discussed further in Chapter 9.

Arterial Pco₂

Measurement

A P_{CO_2} electrode as shown in Figure 2.1 is used. This is essentially a glass pH electrode surrounded by a bicarbonate buffer, which is separated from the blood by a thin membrane through which CO_2 diffuses. The CO_2 alters the pH of the buffer, and this is measured by the electrode, which reads out the P_{CO_2} directly. Calibration is by means of gas with a known P_{CO_2}.

Normal Values

The normal arterial P_{CO_2} is 37–43 mm Hg and is almost unaffected by age. It tends to fall slightly on heavy exercise and to rise slightly during sleep. Sometimes a blood sample obtained by arterial puncture shows a value in the mid 30s. This can be attributed to the acute hyperventilation caused by the procedure and can be recognized by the correspondingly increased pH.

Causes of Increased Arterial Pco₂

There are two major causes of CO_2 retention: hypoventilation and ventilation–perfusion inequality.

Hypoventilation

This was dealt with in some detail earlier in the chapter, where we saw that hypoventilation must cause hypoxemia and CO_2 retention, the latter being more important (Fig. 2.3). The *alveolar ventilation equation*

$$P_{A_{CO_2}} = \frac{\dot{V}_{CO_2}}{\dot{V}_A} \cdot K \qquad \text{(Eq. 2.5)}$$

emphasizes the inverse relationship between the ventilation and the alveolar P_{CO_2}. In normal lungs, the arterial P_{CO_2} closely follows the alveolar value. Whereas the hypoxemia of hypoventilation can be relieved easily by increasing the inspired P_{O_2}, the CO_2 retention can only be treated by increasing the ventilation. This may require mechanical assistance as described in Chapter 10.

Ventilation–Perfusion Inequality

Although this was considered earlier, its relationship to CO_2 retention warrants further brief discussion because of confusion in this area. At one time, it was argued that ventilation–perfusion inequality does not interfere with CO_2 elimination because the overventilated regions make up for the underventilated areas. This is a fallacy, and it is important to realize that ventilation–perfusion inequality reduces the efficiency of transfer of all gases, including, for example, the anesthetic gases.

Why then do we frequently see patients with chronic pulmonary disease and undoubted ventilation–perfusion inequality who have a normal arterial Pco_2? Figure 2.10 shows the usual sequence. The normal relationships between ventilation and blood flow (A) are disturbed by disease, and hypoxemia and CO_2 retention develop (B). However, the chemoreceptors respond to the increased arterial Pco_2 and raise the ventilation to the alveoli. The result is that the arterial Pco_2 is returned to its normal level (C). However, although the arterial Po_2 is somewhat raised by the increased ventilation, it does not return all the way to normal. This can be explained by the shape of the O_2 dissociation curve and, in particular, the strongly depressive action on the arterial Po_2 of lung units with low ventilation–perfusion ratios. Whereas units with high ventilation–perfusion ratios are effective at eliminating CO_2, they have little advantage over normal units in taking up O_2. The end result is that the arterial Pco_2 is effectively lowered to the normal value, but there is relatively little rise in arterial Po_2.

Some patients do not make the transition from stage B to C, or, having made it, revert to B and develop CO_2 retention. What is the reason for this? Generally, these patients have a high work of breathing, often because of a gross increase in airway resistance. Apparently they elect to raise their Pco_2 rather than to expend the extra energy to increase ventilation. It is of interest that if normal subjects are made to breathe through a narrow tube, thus increasing their work of breathing, their alveolar Pco_2 often rises.

We do not fully understand why some patients with ventilation–perfusion inequality increase their ventilation and some do not. As we shall see in Chapter 5, many patients with emphysema hold their Pco_2 at the normal level even

Figure 2.10.   Arterial Po_2 and Pco_2 in different stages of ventilation–perfusion inequality. Initially there must be both a fall in Po_2 and a rise in Pco_2. However, when the ventilation to the alveoli is increased, the Pco_2 returns to normal but the Po_2 remains abnormally low.

when their disease is far advanced. Patients with asthma generally do the same. This can involve a large increase in ventilation to their alveoli. However, other patients, for example, those with severe chronic bronchitis, typically allow their P_{CO_2} to rise much earlier in the course of the disease. It is possible that there is some difference in the central neurogenic control of ventilation in these two groups of patients.

Arterial pH

Measurement

Arterial pH usually is measured with a glass electrode concurrently with the arterial P_{O_2} and P_{CO_2} through the Henderson-Hasselbalch equation:

$$pH = pK + \log \frac{(HCO_3^-)}{0.03\, P_{CO_2}} \qquad (Eq.\ 2.6)$$

where $pK = 6.1$ and (HCO_3^-) is the plasma bicarbonate concentration in millimoles per liter.

Acidosis

This means a decrease in arterial pH or a process that tends to do this. Sometimes the term "acidemia" is used to refer to the actual fall in pH in the blood. Acidosis can be caused by respiratory or metabolic abnormalities, or (frequently) both.

Respiratory Acidosis

This is caused by CO_2 retention, which increases the denominator in the Henderson-Hasselbalch equation and so depresses the pH. Both mechanisms of CO_2 retention, hypoventilation and ventilation–perfusion ratio inequality, can cause respiratory acidosis.

It is important to distinguish between acute and chronic CO_2 retention. A patient with hypoventilation after an overdose of barbiturate is likely to develop acute respiratory acidosis. There is little change in bicarbonate concentration (the numerator in the Henderson-Hasselbalch equation), and the pH therefore falls rapidly as the P_{CO_2} rises. Typically, a doubling of the P_{CO_2} from 40 to 80 mm Hg in such a patient reduces the pH from 7.4 to approximately 7.2.

By contrast, a patient who develops chronic CO_2 retention over a period of many weeks as a result of increasing ventilation–perfusion inequality caused by chronic pulmonary disease typically has a smaller fall in pH. This is because the kidneys retain bicarbonate in response to the increased P_{CO_2} in the renal tubular cells, increasing the numerator in the Henderson-Hasselbalch equation (partially compensated respiratory acidosis).

These relationships are shown diagrammatically in Figure 2.11 (7). Contrast the steep slope of the line for acute CO_2 retention (A) with the shallow slope of the line for chronic hypercapnia (B). Note also that a patient with acute hypoventilation whose P_{CO_2} is maintained over 2 or 3 days moves toward the chronic line as his kidney conserves bicarbonate (point A to C). Conversely, a

Figure 2.11. **Arterial pH–Pco₂ relationships in various types of acid-base distur-bances.** (See text for details.) (Modified from Flenley DC. Another non-logarithmic acid-base diagram? Lancet 1971;1:961–965.)

patient with chronic obstructive pulmonary disease with long-standing CO_2 retention who develops an acute chest infection with worsening of his ventilation–perfusion relationships may move rapidly from point B to C, that is, parallel to line A. However, if he is then artificially ventilated, he may move back to point B, or even beyond.

Metabolic Acidosis

This is caused by a primary fall in the numerator (HCO_3^-) of the Henderson-Hasselbalch equation, an example being diabetic ketoacidosis. Uncompensated metabolic acidosis would be indicated by a vertical upward movement on Figure 2.11, but in practice the fall in arterial pH stimulates the peripheral chemoreceptors, increasing the ventilation and lowering the Pco_2. As a result, the pH and Pco_2 move along line D.

Lactic acidosis is another form of metabolic acidosis, and this may complicate severe acute respiratory or cardiac failure as a consequence of tissue hypoxia. If such a patient is artificially ventilated, the pH remains below 7.4 when the Pco_2 is returned to normal.

Alkalosis (or Alkalemia)

This means an increase in arterial pH.

Respiratory Alkalosis

This is seen in acute hyperventilation where the pH rises, as in E in Figure 2.11. If the hyperventilation is maintained, for example, at high altitude, compensated respiratory alkalosis is seen, with a return of the pH toward normal as the kidney excretes bicarbonate, a movement from E to F.

Metabolic Alkalosis

This is seen in disorders such as severe prolonged vomiting, when the plasma bicarbonate concentration rises, as in G in Figure 2.11. The arterial P_{CO_2} typically increases a little because of slight respiratory depression, although sometimes no change occurs. Metabolic alkalosis also occurs when a patient with long-standing lung disease and compensated respiratory acidosis is ventilated too enthusiastically, thus bringing the P_{CO_2} rapidly to nearly 40 mm Hg (line B to G).

Diffusing Capacity

So far, this chapter on gas exchange has been devoted to arterial blood gases and their significance. However, this is a convenient place to discuss another common test of gas exchange, the diffusing capacity of the lung for carbon monoxide.

Measurement of Diffusing Capacity

The most popular method of measuring the diffusing capacity (Dco) is the single breath method (Fig. 2.12). The patient takes a vital capacity breath of 0.3% CO and 10% helium, holds his or her breath for 10 seconds, and then exhales. The first 750 ml of gas are discarded because of dead space contamination, and

Figure 2.12. Measurement of the diffusing capacity for carbon monoxide by the single breath method. The subject takes a single breath of 0.3% CO with 10% helium, holds his or her breath for 10 seconds, and then exhales. After discarding the first 750 ml, an alveolar sample is collected and analyzed.

the next liter is collected and analyzed. The helium gives the dilution of the inspired gas with alveolar gas and thus gives the initial alveolar Pco. On the assumption that the CO is lost from alveolar gas in proportion to the Pco during breathholding, the diffusing capacity is calculated as the volume of CO taken up per minute per mm Hg alveolar Pco. The diffusing capacity can also be measured by inhaling CO at a low concentration during normal breathing, the so-called steady-state method. (See West JB. Respiratory physiology–the essentials, ed. 5: pp. 26–29 for further details.)

Causes of Reduced Diffusing Capacity

CO is used to measure diffusing capacity because when it is inhaled in low concentrations, the partial pressure in the pulmonary capillary blood remains extremely low in relation to the alveolar value. As a result, CO is taken up by the blood all along the capillary (contrast the time course of O_2 shown in Figure 2.5). Thus, the uptake of CO is determined by the *diffusion properties* of the blood-gas barrier and the *rate of combination* of CO with blood.

The *diffusion properties* of the alveolar membrane depend on its thickness and area. Thus, the diffusing capacity is reduced by diseases in which the thickness is increased, including diffuse interstitial fibrosis, sarcoidosis, and asbestosis (Figure 2.6). It is also reduced when the surface area of the blood-gas barrier is reduced, for example, by pneumonectomy. The fall in diffusing capacity that occurs in emphysema may be caused by the loss of alveolar walls and capillaries (however, see below).

The *rate of combination* of CO with blood is reduced whenever the number of red cells in the capillaries is reduced. This occurs in anemia and also diseases that reduce the capillary blood volume, such as pulmonary embolism. It is possible to separate the membrane and blood component of the diffusing capacity by making the measurement at a high and normal alveolar Po_2.

Interpretation of Diffusing Capacity

In many patients in whom the measured diffusing capacity is low, the interpretation is uncertain. The reason for this is the unevenness of ventilation, blood flow, and diffusion properties throughout the diseased lung. We know that such lungs tend to empty unevenly (Fig. 1.12), so that the liter of expired gas that is analyzed for CO (Figure 2.12) is probably not representative of the whole lung. A reflection of this problem is that different methods of measuring diffusing capacity in patients with diseased lungs frequently show poor agreement.

For this reason, the diffusing capacity is sometimes referred to as the *transfer factor* (especially in Europe) to emphasize that it is more a measure of the lung's overall ability to transfer gas into the blood than a specific test of diffusion characteristics. However, in spite of this uncertainty of interpretation, the test has a definite place in the pulmonary function laboratory and is frequently useful in assessing the severity and type of lung disease.

3

Other Tests

In the first two chapters, we concentrated on two simple but informative tests of pulmonary function: the forced expiration, and arterial blood gases. In this chapter, we briefly consider some of the other ways of measuring lung function. Of the large number of possible tests that have been introduced from time to time, only the most useful are selected, and the principles rather than the details of their use are emphasized.

Static Lung Volumes

Measurement

The measurement of the vital capacity with a simple spirometer was described in Chapter 1 (Fig. 1.1). This equipment can also be used to obtain the tidal volume, inspiratory capacity, and expiratory reserve volume (functional residual capacity minus the residual volume). However, the residual volume, functional residual capacity, and total lung capacity require additional measurements.

The *functional residual capacity* (FRC) can be measured with a body plethysmograph, which is essentially a large airtight box in which the patient sits. (See West JB. Respiratory physiology–the essentials, ed. 5. Baltimore: Williams & Wilkins, 1995:14.) The mouthpiece is obstructed, and the patient is instructed to make rapid panting efforts. As he or she compresses the gas volume in the lungs, the air in the plethysmograph expands slightly and its pressure falls. By applying Boyle's law, the lung volume can be obtained. Another method is to use the helium dilution technique, in which a spirometer of known volume and helium concentration is connected to the patient in a closed circuit. From the degree of dilution of the helium, the unknown lung volume can be calculated. The *residual volume* (RV) can be derived from the FRC by subtracting the expiratory reserve volume.

Interpretation

The FRC and RV often are increased in diseases in which there is an increased airway resistance, for example, emphysema, chronic bronchitis, and asthma. Indeed, at one time, an elevated RV was regarded as an essential feature of emphysema, but less emphasis is placed on this test now. The RV is raised in these conditions because airway closure occurs at an abnormally high lung volume.

A reduced FRC and RV are often seen in patients with reduced lung compliance, for example, in diffuse interstitial fibrosis. Here the lung is stiff and tends to recoil to a smaller resting volume.

If the FRC is measured by both the plethysmographic and gas dilution methods, a comparison of the two results is often informative. The plethysmographic method measures all the gas in the lung. However, the dilution techniques only "see" those regions of lung that communicate with the mouth. Therefore, regions behind closed airways (for example, cysts) result in a higher value for the plethysmographic than for the dilution procedure. The same disparity is often seen in patients with chronic obstructive pulmonary disease, probably because some areas are so poorly ventilated that they do not equilibrate in the time allowed.

Lung Elasticity

Measurement

The pressure-volume curve of the lung requires knowledge of the pressures both in the airways and around the lung. A good estimate of the latter can be obtained from the esophageal pressure. A small balloon on the end of a catheter is passed down through the nose or mouth, and the difference between the mouth and esophageal pressures is recorded as the patient exhales in steps of 1 liter from total lung capacity (TLC) to RV. The resulting pressure–volume curve is not linear (Fig. 3.1), so that a single value for its slope (compliance) is often misleading. However, the compliance is sometimes reported for the liter above FRC measured on the descending limb of the pressure–volume curve.

The pressure-volume curve is often reported using the percentage of predicted TLC on the vertical axis rather than using the actual lung volume in liters (Fig. 3.1) (8). This procedure helps to allow for differences in body size and reduces the variability of the results. Normal values for compliance are given in Appendix A.

Interpretation

Elastic recoil is reduced in patients with emphysema. Figure 3.1 shows that the pressure-volume curve is displaced to the left and has a steeper slope in this condition as a result of the destruction of the alveolar walls (Figs. 4.2, 4.3, and 4.5) and the consequent disorganization of elastic tissue. The change in

Figure 3.1. Pressure-volume curves of the lung. Note that the curves for emphysema and asthma (during bronchospasm) are shifted upward and to the left, whereas those for rheumatic valve disease and interstitial fibrosis are flattened. (From Bates DV, Macklem PT, Christie RV. Respiratory function in disease. 2nd ed. Philadelphia: WB Saunders, 1971.)

compliance is not reversible. The pressure-volume curve is also typically shifted to the left in patients with asthma during an attack, but the change is reversible in some patients. The reasons for this shift are unclear. Increasing age also tends to reduce elastic recoil.

Elastic recoil is increased in interstitial fibrosis, which results in the deposition of fibrous tissue in the alveolar walls (Figs. 2.6 and 5.3), reducing their distensibility. Elastic recoil also tends to increase in patients with rheumatic heart disease who have a raised pulmonary capillary pressure and some interstitial edema. However, it should be noted that measurements of the pressure-volume curve show considerable variability, and the neat results shown in Figure 3.1 are based on the means of many patients.

Airway Resistance

Measurement

Airway resistance is defined as the pressure difference between the alveoli and the mouth divided by the flow rate. Alveolar pressure can only be measured indirectly: one way to do this is with a body plethysmograph. (See West JB. Respiratory physiology–the essentials, ed. 5. Baltimore: Williams & Wilkins, 1995: p. 162.) The subject sits inside an airtight box and pants through a flowmeter. The alveolar pressure can be deduced from the pressure changes in the plethysmograph because, when the alveolar gas is compressed, the plethysmograph gas volume increases slightly, causing a fall in pressure. This method has the great advantage that lung volume can be measured easily almost simultaneously. Figure 3.2 shows the effect of cigarette smoking on airway resistance, here expressed as its reciprocal, *conductance* (9).

Figure 3.2.   Effect of cigarette smoking on airway conductance as measured in the body plethysmograph. The ordinate shows conductance over thoracic gas volume (TGV). (From Nadel JA, Comroe Jr, JH. Acute effects of inhalation of cigarette smoke on airway conductance. J Appl Physiol 1961;16:713–716.)

Other methods of measuring airway resistance are in use. In one, lung volume, flow rate, and esophageal pressure are measured simultaneously. Because tissue resistance is included in this measurement, the result is often called *pulmonary resistance*.

Interpretation

Airway resistance varies inversely with lung volume because the expanding parenchyma exerts traction on the airway walls. Thus, any measurement of airway resistance must be related to the lung volume. Note that the small peripheral airways normally contribute little to overall resistance because there are so many arranged in parallel. For this reason, special tests have been devised to detect early changes in small airways. These changes include the flow rate during the latter part of the flow-volume curve (Fig. 1.8) and closing volume (Fig. 1.11).

Airway resistance is increased in chronic bronchitis and emphysema. In chronic bronchitis, the lumen of a typical airway contains excessive secretions and the wall is thickened by mucous gland hyperplasia and edema (Fig. 4.6). In emphysema, many of the airways lose their support because of destruction of the alveolar walls that surround them (Figs. 4.1 and 4.2). As a result, their resistance may not be increased much during quiet breathing (it may be normal), but with any exertion, dynamic compression (Fig. 1.6) quickly occurs on expiration, and resistance rises strikingly. Such patients often show a reasonably high flow rate early in expiration, but this abruptly drops to low values as flow limitation occurs (see the flow-volume curve in Fig. 1.8). Recall that the driving pressure under these conditions is the static recoil pressure of the lung (Fig. 1.6), which is reduced in emphysema (Fig. 3.1).

Airway resistance is also increased in patients with bronchial asthma. Here the factors include contraction of bronchial smooth muscle with resultant bronchoconstriction, mucous plugs occluding many of the airways, and edema of their walls (Fig. 4.13). The resistance may be high during attacks, especially in relation to lung volume, which is frequently greatly increased. The resistance is reduced by bronchodilator drugs. Even during periods of remission when the patient is asymptomatic, airway resistance is often raised.

Tracheal obstruction causes an increased airway resistance. This may be caused by compression from outside, for example, an enlarged thyroid, or by intrinsic narrowing caused by scarring or a tumor (fixed obstruction). An important feature is that the obstruction is usually apparent during *inspiration* and it can be detected on an inspiratory flow-volume curve (Fig. 1.9). In addition, an audible stridor is often present.

Control of Ventilation

Measurement

The ventilatory response to carbon dioxide can be studied with a rebreathing technique (10). A small bag is filled with a mixture of 6–7% CO_2 in oxygen, and the patient rebreathes from this over a period of several minutes. The bag P_{CO_2} increases at the rate of 4–6 mm Hg/min, and thus the change in ventilation per mm Hg increase in P_{CO_2} can be determined easily.

The ventilatory response to hypoxia can be measured in a similar way. In this instance, the bag is filled with 24% O_2, 7% CO_2, and the balance N_2. During rebreathing, the P_{CO_2} is monitored and held constant by means of a variable bypass and CO_2 absorber. Rebreathing can be continued until the inspired P_{O_2} falls to about 40 mm Hg. This method is technically more difficult than that for the carbon dioxide response and therefore it is used less often.

Both these techniques give information about the overall ventilatory response to CO_2 or hypoxia, but they do not differentiate between patients who *will* not breathe because of central nervous system or neuromuscular inadequacy, and those who *cannot* breathe because of mechanical abnormalities of the chest. To make this distinction between those who "won't" and those who "can't" breathe, the mechanical work done during inspiration can be measured. To accomplish this, the esophageal pressure is recorded together with tidal volume, and the area of the pressure-volume loop is obtained. (See West JB. Respiratory physiology–the essentials, ed. 5. Baltimore: Williams & Wilkins, 1995: p. 115.) Inspiratory work recorded in this way is one useful measure of the neural output of the respiratory center.

Another method of assessing the output of the respiratory center is to measure the inspiratory pressure during a brief period of airway occlusion (11). The patient breathes through a mouthpiece into a valve box that separates the inspired and expired flows, and the inspiratory port is provided with a shutter. This is closed during an expiration (the patient being unaware), so that the first part of the next inspiration is against an occluded airway. The shutter is opened after about ½ second. However, the pressure generated during the first 0.1 second of attempted inspiration ($P_{0.1}$) is taken as a measure of respiratory center output. This is largely unaffected by the mechanical properties of the respiratory system but is influenced by lung volume.

Interpretation

The ventilatory response to CO_2 is depressed by sleep, narcotic drugs, and genetic, racial, and personality factors. An important question is why some patients with chronic pulmonary disease develop CO_2 retention and others do not. In this context, considerable differences of CO_2 response exist between individuals, and it has been suggested that the course of patients with chronic respiratory disease may be related to this factor. Thus, patients who respond strongly to a rise in Pco_2 may be more distressed by dyspnea, whereas those who respond weakly may succumb to respiratory failure.

Figure 3.3A shows the results in three patients with chronic obstructive pulmonary disease who performed an abnormally small amount of inspiratory work in response to inspired CO_2. In addition, they required an inordinately high inspiratory work for a given amount of ventilation (B). Thus, these patients had evidence of both a reduced respiratory center output and mechanical obstruction to breathing (12).

The factors that affect the ventilatory response to hypoxia are less clearly

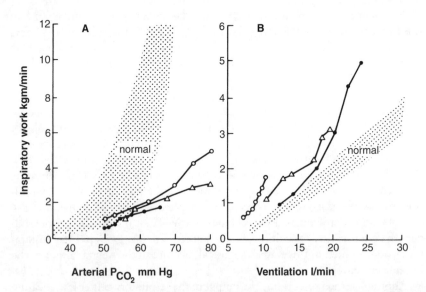

Figure 3.3. Ventilatory response to CO_2 in three patients with chronic obstructive pulmonary disease. *(A)* Shows they performed an abnormally small amount of inspiratory work as the inspired Pco_2 was raised. *(B)* Shows they required an abnormally high work for a given level of ventilation. (From Lane DJ, Howell JBL. Relationship between sensitivity to carbon dioxide and clinical features in patients with chronic airways obstruction. Thorax 1970;25:150–159.)

understood. However, the response is reduced in persons who have been hypoxemic since birth, such as those born at high altitude or with cyanotic congenital heart disease. The hypoxic ventilatory response tends to be preserved during sleep. However, some patients develop sleep apnea syndromes, as discussed on page 21–22.

The $P_{0.1}$ response to occlusion measures the total neural discharge of the respiratory center. Allowance should be made for changes in lung volume because these can affect the relationship between the stimulus to the inspiratory muscles and the pressure that they develop. The $P_{0.1}$ response to occlusion has been shown to be depressed by anesthetics and respiratory depressant drugs.

Exercise Tests

Measurement

The normal lung has enormous reserves of function at rest. For example, the O_2 uptake and CO_2 output can be increased at least 10-fold when a normal subject exercises, and these increases occur without any fall in arterial Po_2 or rise in Pco_2. Therefore, to reveal minor dysfunction, the stress of exercise is often useful.

Another reason for exercise testing is to assess disability. Patients vary considerably in their own assessment of the amount of activity they can do, and an objective measurement on a treadmill or stationary bicycle can be revealing. Occasionally, exercise tests are diagnostic, for example, in exercise-induced asthma or myocardial ischemia causing angina. Exercise tests can help evaluate the cause of dyspnea.

The variables that are often measured during exercise include work load, total ventilation, respiratory frequency, tidal volume, heart rate, ECG, blood pressure, O_2 uptake, CO_2 output, arterial Po_2, Pco_2, and pH. More specialized measurements, such as diffusing capacity, cardiac output, and blood lactate concentration are sometimes made. Abnormal gas exchange can be characterized by the physiologic dead space and shunt as at rest.

Interpretation

In most instances, the interpretation of the tests on exercise is similar to that at rest except that exercise exaggerates the abnormalities. For example, a patient with interstitial lung disease who has a marginally reduced diffusing capacity at rest may show almost no increase on exercise (an abnormal result), with a marked fall in arterial Po_2, a relatively small rise in cardiac output, and perhaps striking dyspnea. Figure 3.4B shows the exercise response of a patient with hypersensitivity pneumonitis (13). Note the rapid increase in ventilation at relatively low work levels and the fall in arterial Po_2 and Pco_2.

Some investigators take special note of the respiratory exchange ratio (R) as the exercise level is increased, although this requires special equipment for its continuous measurement. When the patient reaches the limit of his or her steady-state aerobic exercise *(anaerobic threshold)*, the R rises more rapidly. This

Figure 3.4.   Results obtained during exercise testing. *(A)* Normal pattern. *(B)* Results in a patient with hypersensitivity pneumonitis. Note the restricted work level as evidenced by the limited O_2 intake, the excessive ventilation for the O_2 intake, and the marked fall in arterial Po_2. (From Jones NL. Exercise testing in pulmonary evaluation. N Engl J Med 1975;293:541–544, 647–650.)

is caused by an increase in the CO_2 production secondary to the liberation of lactic acid from the hypoxic muscles. The hydrogen ions react with bicarbonate and lead to an increase in CO_2 excretion above that produced by aerobic metabolism. The fall in pH provides an additional stimulus to breathing.

Sometimes it is possible to identify the chief factor limiting exercise in a patient with mixed disease (14). For example, patients who have both heart and lung disease present a common problem. Exercise testing may reveal that at a patient's maximum work load there is abnormal pulmonary gas exchange with a high physiologic dead space and shunt, suggesting that the patient's lung is the weak link. Alternatively, his or her cardiac output may respond poorly to exercise, thus suggesting heart disease as the chief culprit. Sometimes, however, the interpretation is not clear-cut.

Dyspnea

This is a convenient place to briefly consider one of the most important symptoms of lung disease. *Dyspnea* refers to the sensation of difficulty with breathing, and it should be distinguished from simple tachypnea (rapid breathing) or hyperpnea (increased ventilation). Because dyspnea is a subjective phenomenon, it is difficult to measure, and the factors responsible for it are poorly understood. Broadly speaking, dyspnea occurs when the *demand for ventilation* is out of proportion to the patient's *ability to respond* to that demand. As a result, breathing becomes difficult, uncomfortable, or labored.

An *increased demand for ventilation* is often caused by changes in the blood gases and pH. High ventilations on exercise are commonly seen in patients with inefficient pulmonary gas exchange, especially those with large physiologic dead spaces, who tend to develop CO_2 retention and acidosis unless they achieve high ventilations. Another important factor is stimulation of intrapulmonary receptors. This factor presumably explains the high exercise ventilations in many patients with interstitial lung disease, possibly as a result of stimulation of the juxtacapillary (J) receptors (Figure 3.4B).

A *reduced ability to respond* to the ventilatory needs is generally caused by abnormal mechanics of the lung or chest wall. Frequently, increased airway resistance is the problem, as in asthma, but other causes include a stiff chest wall, as in kyphoscoliosis.

The assessment of dyspnea is difficult. Exercise tolerance often is determined from a standard questionnaire that grades breathlessness according to how far the patient can walk on the level or up stairs without pausing for breath. Occasionally, ventilation is measured at a standard level of exercise and is then related to the patient's maximum voluntary ventilation in an attempt to obtain an index of dyspnea. However, dyspnea is something that only the patient feels; as such, it cannot be measured accurately.

Topographic Differences of Lung Function

Measurement

The regional distribution of blood flow and ventilation in the lung can be measured with radioactive substances. A common method of detecting areas of absent blood flow is by injection of albumin aggregates labeled with radioactive technetium. An image of the radioactivity is then made with a gamma camera, and "cold" areas containing no activity are readily apparent. The major application of this method in practice is the diagnosis of pulmonary embolism.

The distribution of blood flow can also be obtained from an intravenous injection of radioactive xenon or other gas dissolved in saline. When the gas reaches the pulmonary capillaries, it is evolved into the alveolar gas, and the radiation can be detected by a gamma camera. This method has the advantage of giving blood flow per unit volume of lung.

The distribution of ventilation can be measured in a similar way, except that the gas is inhaled into the alveoli from a spirometer. Either a single inspiration or a washin over a series of breaths can be recorded. Again, ventilation per unit volume of lung is available.

Interpretation

The distribution of blood flow in the upright lung is uneven, being much greater at the base than at the apex (Fig. 3.5). The differences are caused by gravity

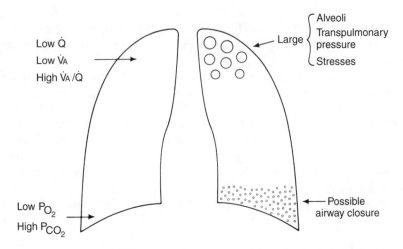

Figure 3.5.   Regional differences of structure and function in the upright lung.

and can be explained by the relationships between the pulmonary arterial, venous, and alveolar pressures. (See West JB. Respiratory physiology–the essentials, ed. 5. Baltimore: Williams & Wilkins, 1995: p. 40.) Exercise results in a more uniform distribution because of the increase in pulmonary arterial pressure, and the same result is found in disease conditions such as pulmonary hypertension and left-to-right cardiac shunts. Increased pulmonary venous pressure, for example, in mitral stenosis, initially causes a more even distribution. However, later in the disease, apical flow may exceed basal flow (Fig. 6.6). The mechanism of this is uncertain, but interstitial edema may play a role. Localized lung disease, for example, a cyst, or area of fibrosis, frequently decreases regional blood flow.

The distribution of ventilation is also gravity-dependent, and normally the ventilation to the base exceeds that to the apex. The explanation is the distortion that the lung suffers because of gravity and the larger transpulmonary pressure at the apex compared with the base. (See West JB. Respiratory physiology–the essentials, ed. 5. Baltimore: Williams & Wilkins, 1995: p. 99.) Localized lung disease, for example, a bulla, usually reduces the ventilation in that area. In generalized lung disease, such as asthma, chronic bronchitis and emphysema, and interstitial fibrosis, areas of reduced ventilation and blood flow can frequently be detected.

Normal subjects show a reversal of the normal pattern of ventilation if they inhale a small amount of radioactive gas from residual volume. The reason is that the airways at the base of the lung are closed under these conditions because intrapleural pressure actually rises above airway pressure. The same pattern may occur at FRC in older subjects because the lower zone airways close at an abnormally high lung volume. Similar findings may be seen in patients with emphysema, interstitial edema, and obesity. All these conditions exaggerate airway closure at the base of the lung.

Other regional differences of structure and function also occur. The gravity-induced distortion of the upright lung causes the alveoli at the apex to be larger than those at the base. These larger alveoli are also associated with greater mechanical stresses that may play a role in the development of some diseases, such as centriacinar emphysema (Figure 4.5A) and spontaneous pneumothorax.

Value of Pulmonary Function Tests

This book is about the function of diseased lungs and it is natural that we should start with a discussion of pulmonary function tests. However, it is important to recognize that these tests have a limited role in clinical practice. They are rarely useful in making a specific diagnosis; rather, they provide supporting information that is added to that obtained from the clinical history, physical examination, chest radiograph, and laboratory tests. Lung function tests are particularly valuable in following the progress of a patient, for example, assessing the efficacy of bronchodilator therapy in a patient with asthma. They also are useful in assessing patients for surgery, determining disability for purposes of worker's compensation, and estimating the prevalence of disease in a community, for example, in a coal mine or an asbestos factory. It is important to appreciate that lung function tests are occasionally within normal limits despite obvious generalized lung disease (Fig. 7.7).

As has been emphasized, spirometry gives useful information with simple equipment. Arterial blood gases are more difficult to measure, but the data may be lifesaving in patients with respiratory failure. The value of the other tests depends to a large extent on the particular clinical problem, and whether they are worth doing is related to the facilities of the pulmonary function laboratory, the expense, and the likelihood that they will give useful information.

Function of the Diseased Lung

This part is devoted to the patterns of abnormal function in the common types of lung disease.

HAROLD BRIDGES LIBRARY
S. MARTIN'S COLLEGE
LANCASTER

4   Obstructive Diseases

Obstructive diseases of the lung are extremely common. In the United States, they are second only to heart disease as a cause of disability benefits under Social Security. They are also becoming increasingly important as a cause of mortality. Unfortunately, as we shall see, the distinctions between the various types of obstructive diseases are blurred, giving rise to difficulties in definition and diagnosis. However, all these diseases are characterized by airway obstruction.

Airway Obstruction

Increased resistance to airflow can be caused by conditions 1) inside the lumen, 2) in the wall of the airway, and 3) in the peribronchial region (Fig. 4.1):

1. The lumen may be partially occluded by excessive secretions, such as in chronic bronchitis. Partial obstruction can also occur acutely in pulmonary edema or after aspiration of foreign material and, postoperatively, with retained secretions. Inhaled foreign bodies may cause localized partial or complete obstruction.
2. Causes in the wall of the airway include contraction of bronchial smooth muscle, as in asthma, hypertrophy of the mucous glands, as in chronic bronchitis (Fig. 4.6), and inflammation and edema of the wall, as in bronchitis and asthma.
3. Outside the airway, destruction of lung parenchyma may cause loss of radial traction and consequent narrowing, as in emphysema. A bronchus may also be compressed locally by an enlarged lymph node or neoplasm. Peribronchial edema can also cause narrowing (Fig. 6.5).

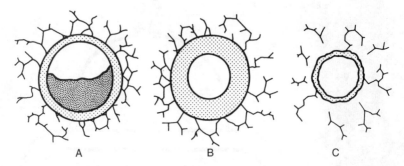

Figure 4.1. Mechanisms of airway obstruction. *(A)* The lumen is partly blocked, for example, by excessive secretions. *(B)* The airway wall is thickened, for example, by edema or muscle hypertrophy. *(C)* The abnormality is outside the airway; in the example shown, the lung parenchyma is partly destroyed and the airway has narrowed because of loss of radial traction.

Chronic Obstructive Pulmonary Disease (COPD)

Chronic obstructive pulmonary disease (COPD) is an ill-defined term that is often applied to patients who have emphysema, chronic bronchitis, or a mixture of the two. There are many patients who report increasing shortness of breath over several years and are found to have a chronic cough, poor exercise tolerance, evidence of airway obstruction, overinflated lungs, and impaired gas exchange. It often is difficult to know to what extent these patients have emphysema or chronic bronchitis, and the term "chronic obstructive pulmonary disease" is a convenient, nondescript label that avoids the necessity of making an unwarranted diagnosis with inadequate data.

Emphysema

Emphysema is characterized by enlargement of the air spaces distal to the terminal bronchiole, with destruction of their walls. Note that this is an anatomic definition; in other words, the diagnosis is presumptive in the living patient.

Pathology

A typical histologic appearance is shown in Figure 4.2B. Note that, in contrast to the normal lung section in Figure 4.2A, the emphysematous lung shows loss of alveolar walls with consequent destruction of parts of the capillary bed (15). Strands of parenchyma that contain blood vessels can sometimes be seen coursing across large dilated air spaces. The small airways (less than 2 mm in diameter) are narrowed, tortuous, and reduced in number. In addition, they have thin, atrophied walls. There is also some loss of larger airways. The structural changes are well seen with the naked eye or hand lens in large slices of lung (Fig. 4.3).

Figure 4.2. Microscopic appearance of emphysematous lung. (*A*) Normal lung. (*B*) Loss of alveolar walls and consequent enlargement of air-spaces (× 90). (From Heard BE. Pathology of chronic bronchitis and emphysema. London: Churchill, 1969.)

Figure 4.3. Appearance of slices of normal and emphysematous lung. (*A*) Normal.
(*B*) Panacinar emphysema (barium sulfate impregnation, $\times$ 14). (From Heard BE. Pathology of
chronic bronchitis and emphysema. London: Churchill, 1969.)

Types

Various types of emphysema are recognized. The definition given above indicates that the disease affects the parenchyma distal to the terminal bronchiole. This unit is the *acinus*, but it may not be damaged uniformly. In *centriacinar emphysema*, the destruction is limited to the central part of the lobule, and the peripheral alveolar ducts and alveoli may escape unscathed (Fig. 4.4). By contrast, *panacinar emphysema* shows distension and destruction of the whole lobule. Occasionally the disease is most marked in the lung adjacent to interlobular septa (*paraseptal emphysema*). In other patients, large cystic areas or bullae develop (*bullous emphysema*).

Centriacinar and panacinar emphysema tend to have different topographic distributions. The former is typically most marked in the apex of the upper lobe but spreads down the lung as the disease progresses (Fig. 4.5A). The predilection for the apex might reflect the higher mechanical stresses (Fig. 3.5), which predispose to structural failure of the alveolar walls. By contrast, panacinar emphysema has no regional preference or, possibly, is more common in the lower lobes. When emphysema is severe, it is difficult to distinguish the two types which may coexist in the same lung. The centriacinar form is extremely common, and mild forms apparently cause no dysfunction.

Another form of emphysema is that associated with α_1-antitrypsin deficiency. Patients who are homozygous for the Z gene frequently develop severe panacinar emphysema, which usually begins in the lower lobes (Fig. 4.5B) (16). The disease may become evident by the age of 40 years and often occurs without cough or smoking history. Therapy by replacement of α_1-antitrypsin is now available. Heterozygotes do not seem to be at risk, although this is not certain. Other variants of emphysema include unilateral emphysema (MacLeod's or Swyer-James syndrome), which causes a unilaterally hyperlucent chest radiograph.

Pathogenesis

This is an active area of research. One current hypothesis is that excessive amounts of the enzyme, lysosomal elastase, are released from the neutrophils in

Figure 4.4. Centriacinar and panacinar emphysema. Note that in centriacinar emphysema, the destruction is confined to the terminal and respiratory bronchioles (TB and RB). In panacinar emphysema the peripheral alveoli (*A*) are also involved.

A

B

the lung. This results in the destruction of elastin, an important structural protein of the lung. Neutrophil elastase also cleaves type IV collagen, and this molecule is important in determining the strength of the thin side of the pulmonary capillary and therefore the integrity of the alveolar wall. Animals that have had neutrophil elastase instilled into their airways develop histologic changes that are similar in many ways to emphysema.

Cigarette smoking is an important pathogenic factor and may work by stimulating macrophages to release neutrophil chemoattractants, such as C5a, or by reducing the activity of elastase inhibitors. In addition, many neutrophils are normally marginated (trapped) in the lung, and this process is exaggerated by cigarette smoking, which also activates trapped leucocytes.

This hypothesis puts the etiology on the same footing as that for the emphysema of α_1-antitrypsin deficiency, in which the mechanism is the lack of the antiprotease that normally inhibits elastase. One puzzle is why some heavy smokers do not develop the disease. Air pollution may play a role, as may hereditary factors, which are clearly important in α_1-antitrypsin deficiency.

Chronic Bronchitis

This disease is characterized by excessive mucus production in the bronchial tree, sufficient to cause excessive expectoration of sputum. Note that this is a clinical definition (unlike the definition of emphysema). In practice, criteria for "excessive" expectoration are often laid down, for example, expectoration on most days for at least 3 months in the year for at least 2 successive years.

Pathology

The hallmark is hypertrophy of mucous glands in the large bronchi (Fig. 4.6) and evidence of chronic inflammatory changes in the small airways (17). The mucous gland enlargement may be expressed as the gland/wall ratio, which is normally less than 0.4 but may exceed 0.7 in severe chronic bronchitis. This is known as the Reid index (Fig. 4.7). Excessive amounts of mucus are found in the airways, and semisolid plugs of mucus may occlude some small bronchi.

In addition, the small airways are narrowed and show inflammatory changes, including cellular infiltration and edema of the walls. Granulation tissue is present and peribronchial fibrosis may develop. Apparently, bronchial smooth muscle increases. There is some evidence that the initial pathologic changes are in the small airways and that these progress to the larger bronchi.

Pathogenesis

Again, cigarette smoking is the chief culprit. Repeated exposure to this inhaled irritant results in chronic inflammation. If you hear a patient give a fruity cough,

---

Figure 4.5. Topographic distribution of emphysema. (*A*) The typical upper zone preference of centriacinar emphysema. (*B*) The typical lower zone preference of emphysema caused by α_1-antitrypsin deficiency. (From Heard BE. Pathology of chronic bronchitis and emphysema. London: Churchill, 1969.)

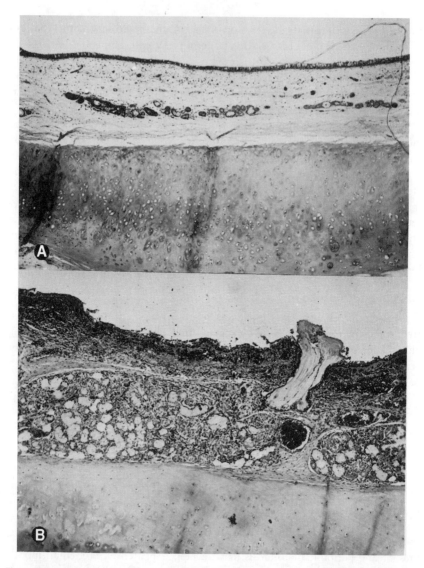

Figure 4.6.   Histologic changes in chronic bronchitis. (*A*) A normal bronchial wall. (*B*) Bronchial wall of a patient with chronic bronchitis. Note the great hypertrophy of the mucous glands, the thickened submucosa, and the cellular infiltration (× 60). Compare with the diagram of the bronchial wall in Figure 4.7. (From Thurlbeck WM. Chronic airflow obstruction in lung disease. Philadelphia: WB Saunders, 1976.)

you can safely bet that he or she is a smoker. Air pollution caused by smog or industrial smoke is another definite factor.

Clinical Features of Chronic Obstructive Pulmonary Disease

As we have seen, chronic bronchitis is a clinical definition, and the diagnosis in the living patient can therefore be made confidently. However, a definitive

Figure 4.7. **Structure of a normal bronchial wall.** In chronic bronchitis, the thickness of the mucous glands increases and can be expressed as the Reid index given by (b–c)/(a–d). (From Thurlbeck WM. Chronic airflow obstruction in lung disease. Philadelphia: WB Saunders, 1976.)

diagnosis of emphysema requires histologic confirmation that is usually not available during life, although a combination of history, physical examination, and radiology (especially computed tomography) can give a high probability of the diagnosis. It follows that the amount of emphysema that is present in a given patient is uncertain; this is why chronic obstructive pulmonary disease remains a useful term.

Within the spectrum of COPD, two extremes of clinical presentation are recognized: type A and type B. At one time it was thought that these types correlated with the relative amounts of emphysema and chronic bronchitis, respectively, in the lung, but the situation is more complicated. Nevertheless, it is still useful to describe two patterns of clinical presentation because they represent different pathophysiologies. In practice, most patients have features of both.

Type A

A typical presentation would be a man in his middle 50s who has had increasing shortness of breath for the last 3 or 4 years. Cough may be absent or may produce little white sputum. Physical examination reveals an asthenic build with evidence of recent weight loss. The chest is overexpanded with quiet breath sounds and no adventitious sounds. The radiograph (Figure 4.8B) confirms the overinflation with low, flat diaphragms, narrow mediastinum, and increased retrosternal translucency (between the sternum and the heart on the lateral view). In addition, the radiograph shows attenuation and narrowing of the peripheral pulmonary vessels. The patients have been dubbed "pink puffers."

Type B

A typical presentation would be a man in his 50s with a history of chronic cough with expectoration for several years. This expectoration has gradually increased in severity, being present only in the winter months initially but, more recently, lasting most of the year. Acute exacerbations with frankly purulent sputum have become more common. Shortness of breath on exertion has gradually worsened, with progressively limiting exercise tolerance. The patient is almost invariably a cigarette smoker of many years' duration.

On examination, the patient has a stocky build with a plethoric complexion and some cyanosis. Auscultation reveals scattered rales and rhonchi. There may be signs of fluid retention with a raised jugular venous pressure and ankle edema. The chest radiograph shows some cardiac enlargement, congested lung fields, and increased markings attributable to old infection. Parallel lines ("tram lines") may be seen, probably caused by the thickened walls of inflamed bronchi. At autopsy, chronic inflammatory changes in the bronchi are the rule if the patient had severe bronchitis, but there may be severe emphysema as well. These patients are sometimes called "blue bloaters."

Pathologic Basis of Types A and B

As indicated earlier, it was initially believed that type A patients predominantly had emphysema while type B patients mainly had chronic bronchitis. However, this notion is too simple (17). Part of the confusion is that different criteria for the two types have been used by different physicians. Naturally, if we restrict the type B classification to patients with severe chronic cough with expectoration, as in the original description (18), such patients are likely to show the pathologic features of chronic bronchitis. However, the extent of the emphysema in the lung is difficult to predict during life.

Some physicians believe that the essential difference between the two types is in the control of breathing. They suggest that the more severe hypoxemia and consequent higher incidence of cor pulmonale in the type B patients can be attributed to a reduced ventilatory drive, especially during sleep.

Pulmonary Function

Most of the features of disordered function in COPD follow from the pathologic features discussed earlier and illustrated in Figures 4.2 to 4.7.

Ventilatory Capacity and Mechanics

The forced expiratory volume in 1 second (FEV_1), vital capacity (FVC), forced expiratory volume as a percentage of vital capacity (FEV/FVC %), forced expi-

---

Figure 4.8. Radiographic appearance in emphysema. (A) Normal lung. (B) The pattern of overinflation, with low flat diaphragms, narrow mediastinum, and increased translucency which is seen in emphysema. The original film also showed attenuation and narrowing of the peripheral pulmonary vessels, but these details do not reproduce well.

ratory flow ($FEF_{25-75\%}$), and maximum expiratory flow at 50% and 75% of exhaled vital capacity ($\dot{V}max_{50\%}$ and $\dot{V}max_{75\%}$) are all reduced. All of these measurements reflect the airway obstruction, whether caused by excessive mucus in the lumen or thickening of the wall by inflammatory changes (Figure 4.1A and B) or by loss of radial traction (Fig. 4.1C). The FVC is reduced because the airways close prematurely at an abnormally high lung volume, giving an increased residual volume (RV). Again, all three mechanisms of Figure 4.1 may be contributing factors.

Examination of the spirogram shows that the flow rate over most of the forced expiration is greatly reduced and the *expiratory time* is much increased. Indeed, some physicians regard this prolonged time as a useful simple bedside index of obstruction. Often, the maneuver is terminated by breathlessness when the patient is still exhaling. The low flow rate over most of the forced expiration partly reflects the reduced elastic recoil of the emphysematous lung, which generates the pressure responsible for flow under these conditions of dynamic compression (Fig. 1.6). Typically, the FEV_1 may be reduced to less than 0.8 liters in severe disease (normal value is approximately 4 liters in young healthy males). Note that the normal values depend on age, height, and sex (see Appendix A).

In some patients, the FEV_1, FVC, and FEV/FVC % may increase significantly after the administration of a bronchodilator aerosol (e.g., 0.5% albuterol by nebulizer for 3 minutes). Such reactive airways are particularly likely to be found in a bronchitic during an exacerbation of infection. Significant response to bronchodilators over a period of weeks suggests asthma, and this disease may overlap with chronic bronchitis ("asthmatic bronchitis").

The expiratory flow-volume curve is grossly abnormal in severe disease. Figure 1.8 shows that, after a brief interval of moderately high flow, flow is strikingly reduced as the airways collapse, and flow limitation by dynamic compression occurs. A scooped-out appearance is often seen. Flow is greatly reduced in relation to lung volume and ceases at a high lung volume because of premature airway closure (Fig. 1.5B). However, the inspiratory flow-volume curve may be normal or nearly so (Fig. 1.9).

The total lung capacity (TLC), functional residual capacity (FRC), and residual volume (RV) are all typically increased in emphysema. Often, the RV/TLC % may exceed 40% (less than 30% in young normals). There is often a striking discrepancy between the FRC determined by the body plethysmograph and the gas dilution techniques (helium equilibration or N_2 washout), the former being higher by 1 liter or more. This may be caused by regions of uncommunicating lung behind grossly distorted airways. However, the disparity more often reflects the slow equilibration process in poorly ventilated areas. These static lung volumes are also often abnormal in chronic bronchitis, although the increases in volume are generally less marked. In COPD, the increased FRC and RV occur because of both the reduced lung elastic recoil and the abnormalities in the airways.

Elastic recoil of the lung is reduced in emphysema (Fig. 3.1), the pressure-volume curve being displaced up and to the left. This change reflects the disorganization and perhaps loss of elastic tissue as a result of destruction of alveolar walls. The transpulmonary pressure at TLC is low. In uncomplicated chronic bronchitis in the absence of emphysema, the pressure-volume curve may be normal because the parenchyma is little affected.

Airway resistance (related to lung volume) is increased in COPD. All the factors shown in Figure 4.1 may be responsible. However, it is possible to distinguish between an increased resistance caused by intrinsic narrowing of the airway or debris in the lumen (Fig. 4.1A and B) and loss of elastic recoil and radial traction (Fig. 4.1C). This can be done by relating resistance to the static elastic recoil (compare Fig. 1.10).

Figure 4.9 shows airway conductance (reciprocal of resistance) plotted against static transpulmonary pressure in a series of 10 healthy patients, 10 patients with emphysema (without bronchitis), and 10 asthmatics (19). The measurements were made during a quiet, unforced expiration. Note that the relationship between conductance and transpulmonary pressure for the patients with emphysema was almost normal. In other words, we can ascribe their reduced ventilatory capacity almost entirely to the effects of the smaller elastic recoil pressure of the lung. This not only reduces the effective driving pressure during a forced expiration but also allows the airways to collapse more easily because of loss of radial traction. The small displacement of the emphysematous line to the right probably reflects the distortion and loss of airways in this disease.

By contrast, the line for the asthmatics shows that the airway conductance was greatly reduced at a given recoil pressure. Thus, the higher resistance in these patients can be ascribed to intrinsic narrowing of the airways caused by

Figure 4.9. Relationships between airway conductance and elastic recoil pressure in obstructive pulmonary disease. Note that the line for emphysema lies close to the normal line. This is evidence that any increase in airway resistance is chiefly caused by the smaller elastic recoil of the lung. By contrast, in asthma, the line is markedly abnormal due to the intrinsic narrowing of the airways. (From Colebatch HJH, Finucane KE, Smith MM. Pulmonary conductance and elastic recoil relationships in asthma and emphysema. J Appl Physiol 1973;34:143–153.)

contraction of smooth muscle and inflammatory changes in the airways. After inhalation of a bronchodilator drug, isoproterenol, the asthmatic line moved toward the normal position (not shown in Fig. 4.9). Comparable data are not available for a group of patients with chronic bronchitis without emphysema because it is virtually impossible to select such a group during life. However, Figure 4.9 clarifies the behavior of different types of airway obstruction.

Gas Exchange

Ventilation–perfusion inequality is inevitable in COPD and leads to hypoxemia with or without CO_2 retention. Typically, the type A patient has only moderate hypoxemia (Po_2 often in the high 60s or 70s) and the arterial Pco_2 is normal. By contrast, the type B patient often has severe hypoxemia (Po_2 often in the 50s or 40s) with an increased Pco_2, especially in advanced disease.

The alveolar-arterial difference for Po_2 is always increased, especially in patients with severe bronchitis. A Riley analysis (Fig. 2.8) reveals increases in both physiologic dead space and physiologic shunt. The dead space is particularly increased in emphysema, whereas high values for shunt are especially common in bronchitis.

The reasons for these differences are clarified by results obtained with the inert gas elimination technique (Fig. 2.9). Figure 4.10 shows a typical distribution in a patient with advanced type A disease (20). This 76-year-old man had a history of increasing dyspnea over several years. The chest radiograph showed hyperinflation with attenuated small pulmonary vessels. The arterial Po_2 and Pco_2 were 68 and 39 mm Hg, respectively.

Figure 4.10. Distribution of ventilation–perfusion ratios in a patient with type A COPD. Note the large amount of ventilation to units with high ventilation–perfusion ratios (physiologic dead space). (From Wagner PD, Dantzker DR, Dueck R, et al. Ventilation–perfusion inequality in chronic pulmonary disease. J Clin Invest 1977;59:203–206.)

The distribution shows that a large amount of ventilation went to lung units with high ventilation–perfusion ratios ($\dot{V}A/\dot{Q}$) (compare Fig. 2.9). This would be shown as physiologic dead space in the Riley analysis and is largely wasted from the point of view of gas exchange. By contrast, there is little blood flow going to units with an abnormally low $\dot{V}A/\dot{Q}$. This explains the relatively mild degree of hypoxemia in the patient and the fact that the calculated physiologic shunt was only slightly increased.

These findings can be contrasted with those shown in Figure 4.11, which shows the distribution in a 47-year-old man with advanced chronic bronchitis and type B disease. He was a heavy smoker and had had a productive cough for many years. The arterial Po_2 and Pco_2 were 47 and 50 mm Hg, respectively. Note that there was some increase in ventilation to high $\dot{V}A/\dot{Q}$ units (physiologic dead space). However, the distribution chiefly shows large amounts of blood flow to low $\dot{V}A/\dot{Q}$ units (physiologic shunt), accounting for his severe hypoxemia. It is remarkable that there was no blood flow to unventilated alveoli (true shunt). Indeed, true shunts of more than a few percent are uncommon in COPD. Note that although the patterns shown in Figures 4.10 and 4.11 are typical, considerable variation is seen in patients with COPD.

On exercise, the arterial Po_2 may fall or rise. The changes depend on the response of the ventilation and the cardiac output, and the changes in distribution of ventilation and blood flow. In some patients at least, the main factor in the fall of Po_2 is the limited cardiac output which, in the presence of ventilation–perfusion inequality, exaggerates any hypoxemia. Patients with CO_2 retention

Figure 4.11. Distribution of ventilation–perfusion ratios in a patient with type B COPD. There is a large amount of blood flow to units with low ventilation–perfusion ratios (physiologic shunt). (From Wagner PD, Dantzker DR, Dueck R, et al. Ventilation–perfusion inequality in chronic pulmonary disease. J Clin Invest 1977;59:203–206.)

often show higher Pco_2 values on exercise because of their limited ventilatory response.

The reasons for the ventilation–perfusion inequality are clear when we consider the disorganization of the lung architecture in emphysema (Figs. 4.2 and 4.3) and the abnormalities in airways in chronic bronchitis (Fig. 4.6). There is ample evidence of uneven ventilation as determined by single breath tests and multibreath washouts. Topographic measurements with radioactive materials show regional inequality of both ventilation and blood flow. The blood flow inequality is largely caused by destruction of portions of the capillary bed. In addition, there is some hypertrophy of smooth muscle in the walls of the small pulmonary arteries in advanced disease, which may contribute to the nonuniformity of flow.

An unresolved question is to what extent the inequality of ventilation in COPD is of the parallel or series type (Fig. 1.11). The essential lesion of centriacinar emphysema is dilatation of the respiratory bronchioles in the middle of the acinus (Fig. 4.4); this is certainly one morphologic abnormality that could cause series inequality. However, we do not yet know how important this mechanism is in practice.

The deleterious effects of airway obstruction on gas exchange are reduced by collateral ventilation that occurs in these patients. Communicating channels normally exist between adjacent alveoli and between neighboring small airways (21), and there have been many experimental demonstrations of these. The fact that there is so little blood flow to unventilated units in these patients (Figs. 4.10 and 4.11) emphasizes the effectiveness of collateral ventilation because some airways must presumably be closed completely, especially in severe bronchitis (Fig. 1.12).

Another factor that reduces the amount of ventilation–perfusion inequality is hypoxic vasoconstriction. (See West JB. Respiratory physiology–the essentials, ed. 5. Baltimore: Williams & Wilkins, 1995: p. 43.) This local response to a low alveolar Po_2 reduces the blood flow to poorly ventilated and unventilated regions, minimizing the arterial hypoxemia. When patients with COPD are given bronchodilators, for example, albuterol, they sometimes develop a slight fall in arterial Po_2. This is probably caused by the vasodilator action of these β-adrenergic drugs, increasing the blood flow to poorly ventilated areas. This finding is more marked in asthma (see later text).

The arterial Pco_2 is often normal in patients with mild to moderate COPD despite their ventilation–perfusion inequality. Any tendency for the arterial Pco_2 to rise stimulates the chemoreceptors, thus increasing ventilation to the alveoli (Fig. 2.10). As disease becomes more severe, the arterial Pco_2 may rise. This is particularly likely to occur in type B patients. The increased work of breathing is an important factor, but there is also evidence that the sensitivity of the respiratory center to CO_2 is reduced in some of these patients (see later text).

If the arterial Pco_2 rises, the pH tends to fall, resulting in respiratory acidosis. In some patients, the Pco_2 rises so slowly that the kidney is able to compensate adequately by retaining bicarbonate, and the pH remains almost constant (compensated respiratory acidosis). In other instances, the P_{CO_2} rises more suddenly, perhaps as a consequence of an acute chest infection. Under these conditions, acute respiratory acidosis may occur (see Chapter 8).

Additional information about gas exchange can be obtained in these patients by measuring the diffusion capacity (transfer factor) for carbon monoxide (Fig. 2.12). The diffusing capacity as measured by the single breath method is particularly likely to be reduced in patients with severe emphysema. By contrast, patients with chronic bronchitis but little parenchymal destruction often have normal values.

These results must be interpreted cautiously. Emphysematous lungs have lost much of their alveolar surface and, thus, the area available for diffusion and the capillary blood volume are reduced. However, it is difficult to know how far the measurement of diffusing capacity reflects this because of the degree of unevenness of ventilation, blood flow, and diffusing properties. Such lungs empty unevenly, and the small post-dead space sample that is analyzed is probably not representative of the lung as a whole. Thus, the diffusing capacity is best regarded as an empirical index of impaired gas transfer with few implications about the morphology of the blood-gas barrier.

Pulmonary Circulation

The pulmonary artery pressure frequently rises in patients with COPD as their disease progresses. Several factors are responsible. In emphysema, large portions of the capillary bed are destroyed, thus increasing vascular resistance. Hypoxic vasoconstriction also raises the pulmonary arterial pressure, and often an exacerbation of chest infection causes an additional transient increase as the hypoxia worsens. Acidosis may exaggerate the hypoxic vasoconstriction. In advanced disease, histologic changes in the walls of the small arteries occur. Finally, these patients often develop polycythemia as a response to the hypoxemia, thus increasing blood viscosity. This occurs most commonly in patients with severe bronchitis who tend to have the lowest arterial P_{O_2}.

Fluid retention with dependent edema and engorged neck veins may occur, especially in type B patients. The right heart often enlarges with characteristic radiologic and electrocardiographic appearances. The term *cor pulmonale* is given to this condition, but whether it should be regarded as right heart failure is disputed. The output of the heart is normally increased because it is operating high on the Starling curve, and the output can rise further on exercise.

Control of Ventilation

As indicated previously, some patients with COPD, particularly those with severe chronic bronchitis, develop CO_2 retention because they do not sufficiently increase the ventilation to their alveoli. The reasons why some patients behave in this way and some do not are not completely understood. One factor is the increased work of breathing as a result of the high airway resistance. As a consequence, the O_2 cost of breathing may be enormous (Fig. 4.12). Normal subjects have an abnormally small ventilatory response to inhaled CO_2 if a

Figure 4.12. Oxygen uptake during voluntary hyperventilation in patients with chronic obstructive lung disease (COLD). Note the high values compared with those of the normal subjects. (From Cherniack RM, Cherniack L, Naimark A. Respiration in health and disease. 2nd ed. Philadelphia: WB Saunders, 1972.)

resistance is attached to the mouthpiece. Thus, a patient with a severely limited O_2 consumption may be willing to forgo a normal arterial Pco_2 to obtain the advantage of a reduced work of breathing and a correspondingly reduced O_2 cost. However, the correlation between airway resistance and arterial Pco_2 is sufficiently poor that some other factor must be involved.

Measurements of the ventilatory response to inhaled CO_2 and of the pressure generated during a brief inspiratory obstruction show that there are significant differences between normal subjects. These differences are partly caused by genetic factors. Some patients can be shown to have a reduced respiratory center output in response to inhaled CO_2, many have a mechanical obstruction to ventilation, and some patients have both (Fig. 3.3). Thus, it is possible that the ventilatory response which a patient makes in the face of severe ventilation–perfusion inequality and increased work of breathing is predetermined to some extent by these factors.

Changes in Early Disease

So far we have mainly been concerned with pulmonary function in patients with well-established disease. However, relatively little can be done to reverse the disease process in this group, and the management is limited chiefly to prevention and control of infection, relief of bronchoconstriction, and general rehabilitative measures. Therefore, there is a great deal of interest in identifying patients with early disease in the hope that the changes can be arrested or reversed. At the very least, these patients could be strongly advised to stop smoking.

It was emphasized in Chapter 1 that, because relatively little of the airway resistance resides in small airways (less than 2 mm diameter), pathophysiologic changes there may go unnoticed by the usual function tests. Some physicians believe that the earliest changes in COPD probably occur in these small airways. Tests of small airway function that are currently being assessed include the FEV_1, $FEF_{25-75\%}$, $\dot{V}max_{50\%}$, and $\dot{V}max_{75\%}$, and closing volume. The practical value of these tests for the early detection of disease is still uncertain.

Management of Patients with COPD

It is critically important that the patient stops smoking but often this is difficult to achieve. Exposure to occupational and atmospheric pollution should be reduced as far as possible. Chronic bronchitis should be treated with antibiotics, and also with bronchodilators if there is a reversible element. Rehabilitation can be helpful in advanced disease.

Recently, lung volume reduction surgery has been reintroduced and is valuable in selected cases, particularly in which there are regions of lung, such as bullae, that are markedly overinflated. The improvement probably occurs by increasing lung elastic recoil, which reduces airway obstruction. The reduced chest volume also improves the efficiency of the respiratory muscles. The long-term benefits of this type of surgery are being evaluated.

Asthma

This disease is characterized by increased responsiveness of the airways to various stimuli and is manifested by widespread narrowing of the airways that changes in severity, either spontaneously or as a result of treatment.

Pathology

The airways have hypertrophied smooth muscle that contracts during an attack, causing bronchoconstriction (Fig. 4.1B). In addition, there is hypertrophy of mucous glands, edema of the bronchial wall, and extensive infiltration by eosinophils (Fig. 4.13). The mucus is abnormal; it is thick, tenacious, and slow-moving.

Normal   **Asthma**

Figure 4.13. Bronchial wall in asthma (diagrammatic). Note the hypertrophied, contracted smooth muscle, edema, mucous gland hypertrophy, and secretion in the lumen.

In severe cases, many of the airways are occluded by mucous plugs, some of which may be coughed up in the sputum. The sputum typically is scant and white. Subepithelial fibrosis is commonly seen in chronic asthma. In uncomplicated asthma, there is no destruction of alveolar walls and there are no copious purulent bronchial secretions. Occasionally, the abundance of eosinophils in the sputum gives a purulent appearance, which may be wrongly ascribed to infection.

Pathogenesis

Rapid progress is being made in this area, and the following account will no doubt be modified. Two features that appear to be common to all asthmatics are airway hyperresponsiveness and airway inflammation. Recent research suggests that the hyperresponsiveness is a consequence of the inflammation, and some investigators believe that airway inflammation is responsible for all the associated features of asthma, including the increased airway responsiveness, airway edema, hypersecretion of mucus, and inflammatory cell infiltration. However, a fundamental abnormality of airway smooth muscle or regulation of airway tone is possible in some patients.

The trigger for the development of airway inflammation cannot always be identified. It is well-recognized in some instances, as in the case for some antigens in allergic asthmatics (Fig. 4.14). However, in other types of asthma, such as exercise-induced asthma or asthma following a viral respiratory tract infection, the trigger is not recognized. Atmospheric pollutants, especially submicronic particles in automobile exhaust gases, may also play a role.

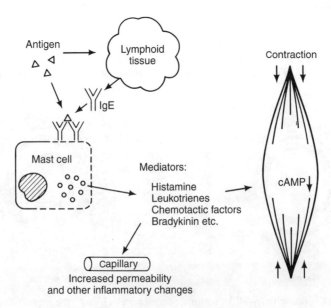

Figure 4.14. Some pathogenic changes in allergic asthma. (See text for details.)

A single inflammatory cell type or inflammatory mediator does not appear to be responsible for all of the manifestations of asthma. Eosinophils, mast cells, neutrophils, macrophages, and basophils have all been implicated. There is also evidence that noninflammatory cells, including airway epithelial cells and neural cells, especially those of peptidergic nerves, contribute to the inflammation. Some investigators believe that eosinophils play a central effector role in most cases of asthma. There is also evidence that lymphocytes, especially T-cells, are implicated, both because they respond to specific antigens and because they have a role as a modulator of inflammatory cell function.

Many inflammatory mediators have been identified in asthma. Cytokines are probably important, particularly those associated with Th-2, helper T-cell activation. These cytokines include granulocyte-macrophage colony-stimulating factor, interleukin (IL)-3, IL-4, and IL-5. It is believed that these cytokines are at least partly responsible for modulating inflammatory and immune cell function, and for supporting the inflammatory response in the airway. Other inflammatory mediators that probably play a role, particularly in acute bronchoconstriction, include arachidonic acid metabolites, such as leukotrienes and prostaglandins, platelet-activating factor (PAF), neuropeptides, reactive oxygen species, kinins, histamine, and adenosine.

Asthma also has a genetic component. Population studies show that it is a complex genetic disorder with both environmental and genetic components. The latter is not a single gene trait but is polygenic. Associations of asthma with a variety of chromosomal loci through linkage analysis has been demonstrated.

Clinical Features

Asthma begins commonly in children but may occur at any age. The patient may have a previous history to suggest atopy, including allergic rhinitis, eczema, or urticaria, and may relate asthmatic attacks to a specific allergen, for example, ragweed or cats. Such a patient is said to have allergic asthma. Many such patients have an increased total serum IgE, increased specific IgE, and peripheral blood eosinophilia. If there is no general history of allergy and no external allergen can be identified, the term nonallergic asthma is used.

In all asthmatics, there is general hyperreactivity of the airways, with the result that nonspecific irritants, such as smoke, cold air, or exercise, cause symptoms. The hyperreactivity (or hyperresponsiveness) of the airways can be tested by exposing the patient to increasing inhaled concentrations of methacholine or histamine and measuring the FEV_1 (or airway resistance). The concentration that results in a 20% fall in FEV_1 is known as the PC_{20} (provocative concentration 20).

Attacks may follow exercise, especially in a cold environment. Aspirin ingestion is a cause in some individuals because of inhibition of the cyclooxygenase pathway. Between attacks, the patient may have no symptoms, although inflammation persists. Psychological factors are important.

During an attack, the patient may be extremely dyspneic, orthopneic, and anxious. The accessory muscles of respiration are active. The lungs are hyperinflated, and musical rhonchi are heard in all areas. The pulse is rapid and pulsus paradoxicus may be present (marked fall in systolic and pulse pressure during inspiration). The sputum is scant and viscid. The chest radiograph reveals hyperinflation but is otherwise normal.

Status asthmaticus refers to an attack that continues for hours or even days without remission despite bronchodilator therapy. There are often signs of exhaustion, dehydration, and marked tachycardia. The chest may become ominously silent, and vigorous treatment is urgently required.

Bronchoactive Drugs

Drugs that reverse or prevent bronchoconstriction play a major role in the management of patients with asthma. They are also useful in those patients with chronic bronchitis who have some reversible airway obstruction.

β-Adrenergic Agonists

β-adrenergic receptors are of two types: β_1 receptors exist in the heart and elsewhere, and their stimulation increases heart rate and the force of contraction of cardiac muscle. Stimulation of β_2 receptors relaxes smooth muscle in the bronchi, blood vessels, and uterus. Partially or completely β_2-selective adrenergic agonists have now completely replaced nonselective agonists. Available drugs include metaproterenol, albuterol, terbutaline, and pirbuterol. These agents have an intermediate duration of action. Long-acting agents, such as salmeterol, have recently become available. All these drugs bind to β_2 receptors in the lung and directly relax airway smooth muscle by increasing the activity of adenyl cyclase, thus raising the intracellular cAMP. They also have effects on airway edema and airway inflammation. Their anti-inflammatory effects are mediated by direct inhibition of inflammatory cell function via binding to β_2 receptors on the cell surface.

These drugs are delivered by aerosol, preferably using a metered-dose inhaler or a nebulizer. Recently, there has been concern about possible tachyphylaxis, particularly in the drug's ability to reverse induced bronchoconstriction when used regularly. Some physicians recommend that they only be used as needed, but the issue is controversial.

Corticosteroids

Corticosteroids appear to have two separate functions: they inhibit the inflammatory/immune response, and they enhance β receptor expression or function. Inhaled corticosteroids are now increasingly used in the management of patients with asthma. However, patients with minimal symptoms that are controlled easily with intermittent β_2 agonists do not require corticosteroids. A wide variety of inhaled corticosteroids are currently available and, when used as directed, result in minimal systemic absorption of corticosteroid with almost no serious side effects. Oral candidiasis and, to a lesser extent, dysphonia may occur with inhaled corticosteroids. Oral corticosteroids are only indicated in patients who do not respond satisfactorily to other aggressive therapies.

Methylxanthines

The mechanism of action of methylxanthines, such as theophylline and amino-phylline, is uncertain. They have modest anti-inflammatory properties and are also bronchodilators, although only about one-fourth as potent as β_2 agonists. The therapeutic dose is close to the toxic dose but they are still useful in the management of chronic asthma. Measurement of blood levels is an aid to developing the correct dose. Aminophylline is sometimes given intravenously during a severe attack of asthma, although its value has been questioned.

Anticholinergics

There is evidence that the parasympathetic nervous system may play a part in the asthma reaction. However, anticholinergics have only a modest bronchodilating effect and only in a subset of asthmatics. By contrast, patients with chronic obstructive pulmonary disease with reversible bronchoconstriction respond more consistently, and anticholinergics are useful here. Ipratropium bromide is the only drug currently available and should be administered as an aerosol.

Cromolyn and Nedocromil

Although these two drugs are structurally unrelated, they apparently have similar mechanisms of action. They were originally thought to be mast cell stabilizers, but it is now recognized that they have broad-ranging effects. They are not direct bronchodilators but presumably work by blocking airway inflammation. Only some patients respond, but when the drugs are effective they can decrease the severity of the disease with virtually no side effects.

New Therapies

This is an active area of research. Leukotriene receptor antagonists and 5-lipoxygenase inhibitors are available, but their role in clinical asthma therapy is unclear so far. There is also research in the areas of phospholipase A_2 inhibitors, phosphodiesterase inhibitors, cytokine antagonists, and antibodies to cytokines.

Pulmonary Function

As was the case with chronic bronchitis and emphysema, the changes in lung function generally follow clearly from the pathology of asthma.

Ventilatory Capacity and Mechanics

During an attack, all indices of expiratory flow rate are reduced significantly, including the FEV_1, FEV/FVC %, $FEF_{25-75\%}$, $\dot{V}max_{50\%}$, and $\dot{V}max_{75\%}$. The FVC is also usually reduced because airways close prematurely toward the end of a full expiration. Between attacks, some impairment of ventilatory capacity can usually be demonstrated although the patient may claim to feel normal.

The response of these indices to bronchodilator drugs is of great importance in asthma (Fig. 4.15). They may be tested by administering 0.5% albuterol by aerosol for 2 minutes. Typically, all indices increase substantially when a bronchodilator is administered to a patient during an attack, and the change is a valuable measure of the responsiveness of the airways. The extent of the increase varies according to the severity of the disease. In status asthmaticus, little change may be seen because the bronchi have become unresponsive. Again, patients in remission may show only minor improvement, although generally there is some.

There is some evidence that the relative change in FEV_1 and FVC after bronchodilator therapy indicates whether the bronchospasm has been completely relived. During an asthma attack, both the FEV_1 and FVC tend to increase by the same fraction, with the result that the FEV/FVC % remains low and almost constant. However, when the tone of the airway muscle is nearly normal, the FEV_1 responds more than the FVC, and the FEV/FVC percent approaches the normal value of approximately 75%.

The flow-volume curve in asthma has the typical obstructive pattern, although it may not exhibit the scooped out appearance seen in emphysema (Fig. 1.8). After a bronchodilator, flows are higher at all lung volumes, and the whole curve may shift as the TLC and RV are reduced.

Static lung volumes are increased, and remarkably high values for FRC and TLC during asthma attacks have been reported. The increased RV is caused by premature airway closure during a full expiration as a result of the increased smooth muscle tone, edema and inflammation of the airway walls, and abnormal secretions. The cause of the increased FRC and TLC is not fully understood. However, there is some loss of elastic recoil, and the pressure-volume curve is shifted upward and to the left (Fig. 3.1). This tends to return toward normal

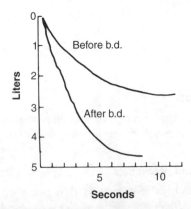

Figure 4.15.   Examples of forced expirations before and after bronchodilator (b.d.) therapy in a patient with bronchial asthma. Note the striking increase in flow rate and vital capacity. (From Bates DV, Macklem PT, and Christie RV. Respiratory function in disease ed 2 Philadelphia, WB Saunders, 1971).

after a bronchodilator. There is some evidence that changes in the surface tension of the alveolar lining layer may be responsible for the altered elastic properties. The rise in lung volume tends to decrease resistance of the airways by increasing their radial traction. The FRC measured by helium dilution is usually considerably below that found with the body plethysmograph, reflecting the presence of occluded airways or the delayed equilibration of poorly ventilated areas.

Airway resistance as measured in the body plethysmograph is raised, and it falls after a bronchodilator. It is likely that the bronchospasm affects airways of all sizes, and the relationship between airway conductance and elastic recoil pressure is significantly abnormal (Fig. 4.9). Narrowing of the large and medium-sized bronchi can be seen directly at bronchoscopy.

Gas Exchange

Arterial hypoxemia is common in asthma and is caused by ventilation–perfusion ($\dot{V}A/\dot{Q}$) inequality. There is ample evidence of uneven ventilation, and measurements with radioactive gases show regions of reduced ventilation. Marked topographical inequality of blood flow is also seen and, typically, different areas show transient reductions at different times. Both physiologic dead space and physiological shunt are generally abnormally high.

An example of a distribution of ventilation–perfusion ratios in a 47-year-old asthmatic is shown in Figure 4.16. This patient had only mild symptoms at the time of the measurement. The distribution is strikingly different from the normal distribution shown in Figure 2.9. Note especially the bimodal distribution with

Figure 4.16. Distribution of ventilation–perfusion ratios in a patient with asthma.
Note the bimodal appearance, with approximately 25% of the total blood flow going to units with ventilation–perfusion ratios in the region of 0.1.

a considerable amount of the total blood flow (approximately 25%) going to units with a low $\dot{V}A/\dot{Q}$ (approximately 0.1). This accounts for the patient's mild hypoxemia, the arterial Po_2 being 81 mm Hg. There is no pure shunt (blood flow to unventilated alveoli), a surprising finding in view of the mucous plugging of airways, which is a feature of the disease.

When this patient was given the bronchodilator isoproterenol by aerosol, there was an increase in $FEF_{25-75\%}$ from 3.4 to 4.2 liters/sec. Thus, there was some relief to his bronchospasm. The changes in the distribution of ventilation–perfusion ratios are shown in Figure 4.17. Note that the blood flow to the low $\dot{V}A/\dot{Q}$ alveoli increased from approximately 25 to 50% of the total flow, resulting in a fall in arterial Po_2 from 81 to 70 mm Hg. The mean $\dot{V}A/\dot{Q}$ of the low mode increased slightly from 0.10 to 0.14, indicating that the ventilation to these units increased slightly more than their blood flow. Again no shunt was seen.

Many bronchodilators, including isoproterenol, aminophylline, and terbutaline, decrease the arterial Po_2 in asthmatics. The mechanism of the increased hypoxemia is apparently relief of vasoconstriction in poorly ventilated areas. This vasoconstriction probably results from the release of mediators, like the bronchoconstriction. The fall in Po_2 is accompanied by increases in physiologic shunt and dead space. However, in practice, the favorable effects of the drugs on airway resistance far exceed the disadvantages of the mild additional hypoxemia.

The absence of shunt–that is, blood flow to unventilated lung units–in Figures 4.16 and 4.17 is striking, especially because asthmatics who come to autopsy have mucous plugs in many of their airways. Presumably, the explanation is collateral ventilation that reaches lung situated behind completely closed bron-

Figure 4.17. The same patient as in Figure 4.16 after the administration of the bronchodilator isoproterenol by aerosol. Note the increase in blood flow to the units with low ventilation–perfusion ratios and the corresponding fall in arterial Po_2.

chioles. This is shown diagrammatically in Figure 1.12. The same mechanism probably exists in the lungs of patients with chronic bronchitis (see Fig. 4.11 for example).

The arterial Pco_2 in patients with asthma is typically normal or low, at least until late in the disease. The Pco_2 is prevented from rising by increased ventilation to the alveoli in the face of the ventilation–perfusion inequality (compare Fig. 2.10). In many patients, the Pco_2 may be in the middle or low 30s, possibly as a result of stimulation of the peripheral chemoreceptors by the mild hypoxemia or stimulation of intrapulmonary receptors.

In status asthmaticus, the arterial Pco_2 may begin to rise and the pH to fall. This is an ominous development that denotes impending respiratory failure and signals the need for urgent and intensive treatment. Mechanical ventilation may be necessary (Chapter 10). Deaths from asthma have apparently increased in recent years and respiratory failure is one cause. Another cause may be overuse of β-adrenergic drugs by inhalers. However, some severe asthmatics are undertreated because the dangers of their disease are not appreciated sufficiently.

The diffusing capacity for carbon monoxide is typically normal or high in uncomplicated asthma. If it is reduced, associated emphysema should be suspected. The reason for the increased diffusing capacity is probably the large lung volume. Hyperinflation increases the diffusing capacity in normal subjects, presumably by increasing the area of the blood-gas interface.

Localized Airway Obstruction

So far, this chapter has been devoted to generalized airway obstruction, both irreversible, as in emphysema and chronic bronchitis, and reversible, as in asthma. (Some patients with chronic bronchitis may show some reversibility.) Localized obstruction is less common and generally causes less functional impairment. Obstruction may be within the lumen of the airway, in the wall, or as a result of compression from outside the wall (Fig. 4.1).

Tracheal Obstruction

This can be caused by an inhaled foreign body, stenosis after the use of an indwelling tracheostomy tube, or compressing masses, such as an enlarged thyroid. There is inspiratory and expiratory stridor, abnormal inspiratory and expiratory flow-volume curves (Fig. 1.9), and no response to bronchodilators. Hypoventilation may result in hypercapnia and hypoxemia (Fig. 2.3).

Bronchial Obstruction

This is often caused by a foreign body, for example, an inhaled peanut. The right lung is more frequently affected than the left because the left main bronchus makes a sharper angle with the trachea than does the right. Other common causes are bronchial tumors, either malignant or benign, and compression of a bronchus by enlarged surrounding lymph nodes. This last cause particularly affects the right middle lobe bronchus because of its anatomic relationships.

If obstruction is complete, absorption atelectasis occurs because the sum of the partial pressures in mixed venous blood is less than in alveolar gas. (See West JB. Respiratory physiology—the essentials, ed. 5. Baltimore: Williams & Wilkins, 1995: p. 141.) The collapsed lobe is often visible on the radiograph, and compensatory overinflation of adjacent lung and displacement of a fissure may also be seen. Perfusion of the unventilated lung is reduced because of hypoxic vasoconstriction and also the increased vascular resistance caused by the mechanical effects of the reduced volume on the extra-alveolar vessels and the capillaries. However, the residual blood flow contributes to hypoxemia. The most sensitive test is the alveolar-arterial Po_2 difference during 100% O_2 breathing (Fig. 2.7). Infection may follow localized obstruction and lead to lung abscess. If the obstruction is in a segmental or smaller bronchus, atelectasis may not occur because of collateral ventilation (Fig. 1.12).

5

Restrictive Diseases

Restrictive diseases are those in which the expansion of the lung is restricted either because of alterations in the lung parenchyma or because of disease of the pleura, the chest wall, or the neuromuscular apparatus. They are characterized by a reduced vital capacity and a small resting lung volume (usually), but the airway resistance (related to lung volume) is not increased. These diseases are therefore different from the obstructive diseases in their pure form, although mixed restrictive and obstructive conditions can occur.

Diseases of the Lung Parenchyma

This term refers to the alveolar tissue of the lung. A brief review of the structure of this tissue is pertinent.

Structure of the Alveolar Wall

Figure 5.1 shows an electron micrograph of a pulmonary capillary in an alveolar wall (25). The various structures through which oxygen passes on its way from the alveolar gas to the hemoglobin of the red blood cell are pulmonary surfactant (not shown in this preparation), alveolar epithelium, interstitium, capillary endothelium, plasma, and erythrocyte.

Cell Types

The various cell types have different functions and different responses to injury.

Type I Epithelial Cell

This is the chief structural cell of the alveolar wall; its long protoplasmic extensions pave almost the whole alveolar surface (Fig. 5.1). The main function of

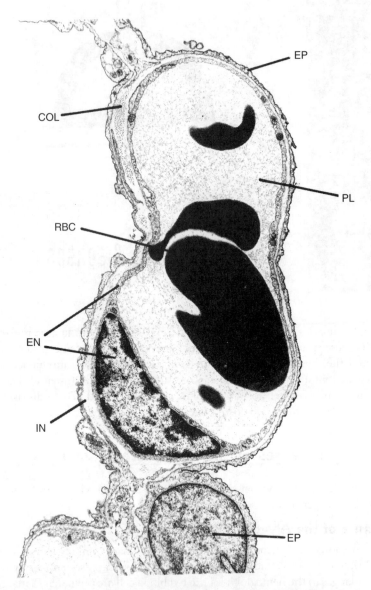

Figure 5.1.   Electron micrograph of portion of an alveolar wall. *EP*, epithelium; *COL*, collagen; *PL*, plasma; *RBC*, red blood cell; *EN*, endothelial cell; *IN*, interstitium (× 6300). (From Weibel ER. Morphological basis of alveolar-capillary gas exchange. Physiol Rev 1973; 53:419–495.)

this cell is mechanical support. It rarely divides and is not very active metabolically. When type 1 cells are injured, they are replaced by type 2 cells, which
later transform into type 1.

Type 2 Epithelial Cell

This is a nearly globular cell (Fig. 5.2) (26) that gives little structural support
to the alveolar wall but is metabolically active. The electron micrograph shows
the lamellated bodies that contain phospholipid. This is formed in the endoplas-
mic reticulum, passed through the Golgi apparatus, and eventually extruded into

Figure 5.2. Electron micrograph of type 2 epithelial cell (× 10,000). Note the lamellated
bodies *(LB)*, large nucleus, and microvilli *(arrows)*, which are mainly concentrated around the
edge of the cell, and cytoplasm rich in organelles. The *inset at top right* is a scanning electron
micrograph showing the surface view of a type 2 cell with its characteristic distribution of
microvilli (× 3400). (From Weibel ER, Gil J. Structure-function relationships at the alveolar level.
In: West JB. ed. Bioengineering aspects of the lung. New York: Marcel Dekker, 1977.)

the alveolar space to form surfactant. (See West JB. Respiratory physiology–the essentials, ed. 5. Baltimore: Williams & Wilkins, 1995: p. 95.) After injury to the alveolar wall, these cells rapidly divide to line the surface and then later transform into type 1 cells. A type 3 cell has also been described, but it is rare and its function is unknown.

Alveolar Macrophage

This scavenger cell roams around the alveolar wall phagocytosing foreign particles and bacteria. The cell contains lysozymes that digest engulfed foreign matter.

Fibroblast

This cell synthesizes collagen and elastin, which are components of the interstitium of the alveolar wall. After various disease insults, large amounts of these materials may be laid down. This results in interstitial fibrosis.

Interstitium

This fills the space between the alveolar epithelium and the capillary endothelium. Figure 5.1 shows that it is thin on one side of the capillary, where it consists only of the fused basement membranes of the epithelial and endothelial layers. On the other side of the capillary, the interstitium is usually wider and includes fibrils of collagen. The thick side is chiefly concerned with fluid exchange across the endothelium, whereas the thin side is responsible for most of the gas exchange (Fig. 6.1).

Interstitial tissue is found elsewhere in the lung, notably in the perivascular and peribronchial spaces around the larger blood vessels and airways and in the interlobular septa. The interstitium of the alveolar wall is continuous with that in the perivascular spaces (Fig. 6.1) and is the route by which fluid drains from the capillaries to the lymphatics.

Diffuse Interstitial Pulmonary Fibrosis

The nomenclature of this condition is confusing. Synonyms include idiopathic pulmonary fibrosis, interstitial pneumonia, and cryptogenic fibrosing alveolitis. Some physicians reserve the term "fibrosis" for the late stages of the disease. The changes in pulmonary function are described in detail because they are typical of many of the other conditions alluded to later in this chapter.

Pathology

The principal feature is thickening of the interstitium of the alveolar wall. Initially there is infiltration with lymphocytes and plasma cells. Later, fibroblasts appear and lay down thick collagen bundles (Fig. 5.3) (27). These changes may be dispersed irregularly within the lung. In some patients, a cellular exudate consisting of macrophages and other mononuclear cells is seen within the alveoli in the early stages of the disease. This is called "desquamation." Eventually, the alveolar architecture is destroyed and the scarring results in multiple air-filled

Figure 5.3.   Electron micrograph from a patient with diffuse interstitial fibrosis. Note the thick bundles of collagen. *COL*, collagen; *ALV*, alveolar space; *RBC*, red blood cell; *PL*, plasma. Compare Figure 5.1. (From Gracey DR, Divertie MD, Brown AL, Jr. Alveolar-capillary membrane in idiopathic interstitial pulmonary fibrosis. Electron microscopic study of 14 cases. Am Rev Respir Dis 1968;98:16–21.)

cystic spaces formed by dilated terminal and respiratory bronchioles–so-called "honeycomb lung."

Etiology

Etiology is unknown, although in some cases there is evidence of an immunologic reaction.

Clinical Features

The disease is not common and tends to affect adults in late middle age. The patient often presents with dyspnea with rapid, shallow breathing. The dyspnea typically becomes significant on exercise (compare Fig. 3.4). An irritating, unproductive cough is often present.

On examination, cyanosis may be seen at rest in severe cases. It typically worsens on exercise. Fine crepitations are usually heard throughout both lungs, especially toward the end of inspiration. Finger clubbing is common. The chest radiograph shows a reticular or reticulonodular pattern, especially at the bases. Patchy shadows near the diaphragm may be caused by basal collapse. Late in the disease, a honeycomb appearance is often seen; this is caused by multiple air cysts surrounded by thickened tissue.

Cor pulmonale or pneumonia may complicate the picture, and the patient may develop respiratory failure terminally. The diseases often progress insidiously, although an acute form occurs as originally described by Hamman and Rich (28).

Pulmonary Function

Ventilatory Capacity and Mechanics

Spirometry typically reveals a restrictive pattern (Fig. 1.2). The FVC is markedly reduced but the gas is exhaled rapidly so that, although the FEV_1 is low, the FEV/FVC percent may exceed the normal value. The almost square shape of the forced expiratory spirogram is in striking contrast to the obstructive pattern (compare Fig. 4.15). The $FEF_{25-75\%}$ is normal or high. The flow-volume curve does not show the scooped-out shape of obstructive disease, and the flow rate is often higher than normal when related to absolute lung volume. This is shown in Figure 1.5 where it can be seen that the downslope of the curve for restrictive disease lies above the normal curve.

All lung volumes are reduced, including the TLC, FRC, and RV, but the relative proportions are more or less preserved. The pressure-volume curve of the lung is flattened and displaced downward (Fig. 3.1), so that at any given volume, the transpulmonary pressure is abnormally high. The maximum elastic recoil pressure that can be generated at TLC is typically higher than normal. Airway resistance is normal or low when related to lung volume.

All these results are consistent with the pathologic appearance of fibrosis of the alveolar walls (Figs. 2.6 and 5.3). The fibrous tissue reduces the distensibility of the lung just as a scar on the skin reduces its extensibility. As a result, the lung volumes are small, and abnormally large pressures are required to distend the lung. The airways may not be specifically involved, but they tend to narrow as lung volume is reduced. However, airway resistance at a given lung volume is normal or even decreased because the retractile forces exerted on the airway walls by the surrounding parenchyma are abnormally high (Fig. 5.4). The pathologic correlate of this is the honeycomb appearance caused by the dilated terminal and respiratory bronchioles surrounded by thickened scar tissue.

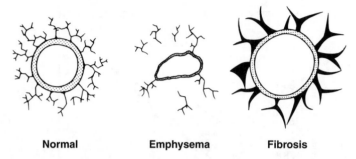

Normal   **Emphysema**   **Fibrosis**

Figure 5.4. Airway caliber in emphysema and interstitial fibrosis. In emphysema, the airways tend to collapse because of the loss of radial traction. By contrast, in fibrosis, radial traction may be excessive, with the result that airway caliber is large when related to lung volume.

Gas Exchange

The arterial Po_2 and Pco_2 are typically reduced and the pH is normal. The hypoxemia is usually mild at rest until the disease is advanced. However, on exercise, the Po_2 often falls dramatically and cyanosis may be evident. In well-established disease, both the physiologic dead space and physiologic shunt are increased.

The relative contribution of diffusion impairment and ventilation–perfusion ($\dot{V}A/\dot{Q}$) inequality to the hypoxemia of these patients has long been debated. It is natural to argue that the histologic appearances shown in Figures 2.6 and 5.3 slow the diffusion of oxygen from the alveolar gas to the capillary blood because the thickness of the barrier may be increased many fold (compare Fig. 5.1). In addition, the increasing hypoxemia on exercise is consistent with the mechanism of impaired diffusion because exercise reduces the time spent by the red cell in the pulmonary capillary (Fig. 2.5).

However, we now know that impaired diffusion is not the chief cause of the hypoxemia in these conditions. First, the normal lung has enormous reserves of diffusion in that the Po_2 of the blood nearly reaches that in alveolar gas early in its transit through the capillary (Fig. 2.5). In addition, these patients have substantial inequality of ventilation and blood flow within the lung. How could they not, with the disorganization of architecture shown in Figures 2.6 and 5.3? The inequalities have been demonstrated by single breath and multibreath N_2 washouts and measurements of topographical function with radioactive gases.

To apportion blame for the hypoxemia between the two possible mechanisms, it is necessary to measure the degree of $\dot{V}A/\dot{Q}$ inequality and determine how much of the hypoxemia is attributable to this. This has been done by using the multiple inert gas elimination technique in a series of patients with interstitial lung disease (29). Figure 5.5 shows that at rest, the hypoxemia could be adequately explained by the degree of $\dot{V}A/\dot{Q}$ inequality present in these patients. However, Figure 5.6 shows that on exercise, the observed alveolar Po_2 was consistently below the value predicted from the measured amount of $\dot{V}A/\dot{Q}$ inequality, and

Figure 5.5. Study of the mechanism of hypoxemia in a series of patients with interstitial lung disease. This figure shows that the arterial Po_2 predicted from the pattern of $\dot{V}A/\dot{Q}$ inequality agreed well with the measured arterial Po_2. Thus at rest, all of the hypoxemia could be explained by the uneven ventilation and blood flow.

Figure 5.6. Results obtained on exercise in the same patients as shown in Figure 5.5. Note that under these conditions the measured arterial Po_2 was systematically below that predicted from the pattern of $\dot{V}A/\dot{Q}$ inequality. This indicates an additional mechanism for hypoxemia, presumably diffusion impairment.

thus an additional cause of hypoxemia must have been present. Most likely this was diffusion impairment in these patients. However, hypoxemia caused by diffusion impairment was only evident on exercise, and even then it accounted for only about one-third of the total alveolar-arterial difference for P_{O_2}.

The low arterial P_{CO_2} in these patients (typically in the middle or low 30s) occurs despite the evident $\dot{V}_A/\dot{Q}$ inequality and is caused by increased ventilation to the alveoli (compare Fig. 2.10). The cause of the increased ventilation is uncertain. There is some evidence that the control of ventilation is abnormal because of stimulation of receptors within the lung (see later text). Stimulation of the peripheral chemoreceptors by the arterial hypoxemia may also be a factor. The arterial pH is usually normal at rest but may increase considerably on exercise as a result of the hyperventilation and consequent respiratory alkalosis (compare Fig. 3.4), although metabolic acidosis caused by lactic acid accumulation may also occur. In terminal respiratory failure, the pH may fall.

The diffusing capacity for carbon monoxide is often strikingly reduced in these patients to the neighborhood of 5 ml/min/mm Hg (normal value near 30 depending on age and stature). This may be a useful diagnostic pointer: if the diffusing capacity is not low, the diagnosis should be regarded with suspicion. The reduction is caused in part by the thickening of the blood-gas barrier (Fig. 2.6). In addition, the blood volume of the pulmonary capillaries decreases because many of the vessels are obliterated by the fibrotic process. A further factor in the lower measured diffusing capacity is probably the $\dot{V}_A/\dot{Q}$ inequality, which causes uneven emptying of the lung. The diffusing capacity should not be taken to reflect only the properties of the blood-gas barrier.

Exercise

Patients with mild diffuse interstitial fibrosis may show much more evidence of impaired pulmonary function on exercise than at rest. The changes shown in Figure 3.4B are typical, although this patient had hypersensitivity pneumonitis (see later text). Note that the maximal O_2 intake and CO_2 output were severely limited compared with the normal values of Figure 3.4A. The increase in ventilation on exercise was greatly exaggerated. This exaggeration was chiefly caused by the high rate of breathing, which rose to over 60 breaths/minute during maximal exercise.

As a result of the high ventilation, which was out of proportion to the increase in O_2 uptake and CO_2 output, the alveolar and arterial P_{CO_2} fell and the alveolar P_{O_2} rose. However, the arterial P_{O_2} fell as noted earlier, thus increasing the alveolar-arterial difference for P_{O_2}. This result can be explained partly by the impaired diffusion characteristics of the lung (Fig. 5.6). However, most of the hypoxemia on exercise was caused by $\dot{V}_A/\dot{Q}$ inequality.

One factor that tends to reduce the arterial P_{O_2} on exercise is the abnormally small rise in cardiac output. These patients typically have an increased pulmonary vascular resistance. This is particularly evident on exercise, during which the pulmonary artery pressure may rise substantially. The high resistance can be attributed to obliteration of much of the pulmonary capillary bed by the interstitial fibrosis (Fig. 2.7). Another factor is hypertrophy of vascular smooth muscle and consequent narrowing of the small arteries. It is important to appreciate that an abnormally low cardiac output in the presence of $\dot{V}A/\dot{Q}$ inequality can cause hypoxemia. One way of looking at this is that a low cardiac output results in a low Po_2 in the mixed venous blood (Chapter 9). As a consequence, a lung unit with a given $\dot{V}A/\dot{Q}$ will oxygenate the blood less than when the mixed venous Po_2 is normal.

The importance of this factor can be seen if we consider some results obtained in our laboratory in a patient with interstitial lung disease. During exercise which raised the O_2 uptake from about 300 to 700 ml/min, the arterial Po_2 fell from 50 to 35 mm Hg. The rise in cardiac output was only from 4.6 to 5.7 liters/min; the normal value for this level of exercise is approximately 10 liters/min. As a result, the Po_2 in the mixed venous blood fell to 17 mm Hg (normal value is approximately 35 mm Hg). Calculations show that if the cardiac output had increased to 10 liters/min (and the pattern of $\dot{V}A/\dot{Q}$ inequality remained unchanged), the arterial Po_2 would have been some 10 mm Hg higher.

If the diffusing capacity for carbon monoxide is measured in these patients during exercise, it typically remains low, whereas it may double or triple in normal subjects. These measurements must be made by the steady state rather than the single breath method because of the difficulties of breath-holding during exercise. This measurement is now seldom done.

Control of Ventilation

We have already seen that these patients typically have shallow rapid breathing, especially on exercise. The reason for this is not known, but it is possible that the pattern is caused by reflexes originating in pulmonary irritant receptors or J (juxtacapillary) receptors. The former lie in the bronchi or in the epithelial lining and may be stimulated by the increased traction on the airways caused by the increased elastic recoil of the lung (Fig. 5.4). The J receptors are in the alveolar walls and could be stimulated by the fibrotic changes in the interstitium. No direct evidence of increased activity of either receptor is yet available in humans, but work in experimental animals suggests that they could cause rapid shallow breathing.

The rapid shallow pattern of breathing reduces the respiratory work in patients with a reduced lung compliance. However, it also increases ventilation of the anatomic dead space at the expense of the alveoli so a compromise must be reached.

Other Types of Parenchymal Restrictive Disease

The changes in pulmonary function in diffuse interstitial pulmonary fibrosis were dealt with at some length because this disease serves as a prototype for other forms of parenchymal restrictive disease. These diseases are now considered briefly here, and differences in their pattern of pulmonary function are discussed.

Sarcoidosis

This disease is characterized by the presence of granulomatous tissue having a characteristic histologic appearance. It often occurs in several organs.

Figure 5.7. Chest radiograph of a patient with interstitial pulmonary fibrosis. Note the small contracted lung and rib cage and the raised diaphragms (compare the normal appearance in Figure 4.8*A*).

Pathology

The characteristic lesion is the noncaseating epithelioid granuloma composed of large histiocytes with giant cells and lymphocytes. This lesion may occur in the lymph nodes, lungs, skin, eyes, liver, spleen, and elsewhere. In advanced pulmonary disease, fibrotic changes in the alveolar walls are seen.

Etiology

Etiology is unknown, although an immunologic basis appears likely. One possibility is that an unknown antigen is recognized by an alveolar macrophage, and this results in activation of a T lymphocyte and the production of interleukin-2. The activated macrophage may also release various products that stimulate fibroblasts, thus explaining the deposition of fibrous tissue in the interstitium.

Clinical Features

Four stages can be identified (30). *Stage 0:* These patients have no obvious intrathoracic involvement, although a CT scan may show enlarged mediastinal lymph nodes (lymphadenopathy). *Stage 1:* There is bilateral hilar adenopathy often with right paratracheal adenopathy. This is often accompanied by erythema nodosum of the legs. Arthritis, uveitis, and parotic gland enlargement may also occur. There are no disturbances of pulmonary function. *Stage 2:* The pulmonary parenchyma is also involved, the most common radiologic appearance being widespread mottled shadows, most significant in the mid and upper zones. Symptoms include breathlessness and a dry, unproductive cough. *Stage 3:* Here there are pulmonary infiltrates without adenopathy. Fibrosis is seen predominantly in the upper lobes, and cavities or bullae may be present.

Pulmonary Function

There is no impairment of function in Stages 0 and 1 of the disease. In Stages 2 and 3, typical changes of the restrictive type are seen, although the radiographic appearance sometimes suggests more interference with function than actually exists.

Ultimately, significant pulmonary fibrosis may develop, with a severe restrictive pattern of function. All lung volumes are small, but the FEV/ FVC% is preserved. Lung compliance is strikingly reduced, the pressure-volume curve being flattened and shifted downward and to the right (Fig. 3.1). The resting arterial Po_2 is low and often falls considerably on exercise. The arterial Pco_2 is normal or low, although, terminally, it may rise as respiratory failure supervenes. The diffusing capacity for carbon monoxide (transfer factor) is reduced significantly. Cor pulmonale may develop in advanced disease.

Hypersensitivity Pneumonitis

This is also known as extrinsic allergic alveolitis. It is a hypersensitivity reaction affecting the lung parenchyma that occurs in response to inhaled organic dusts. A good example is farmer's lung. The exposure is usually occupational and heavy. The disease is an example of type 3 hypersensitivity (or combination of type 3 and type 4), and precipitins can be demonstrated in the serum.

The term "extrinsic" implies that the etiologic agent is external and can be identified, in contrast to "intrinsic" fibrosing alveolitis (diffuse interstitial fibrosis discussed above), where the cause is unknown. Farmer's lung is due to the spores of thermophilic *Actinomyces* in moldy hay. Bird breeder's lung is caused by avian antigens from feathers and excreta. Air conditioner's lung and bagassosis (in sugar cane workers) are also recognized.

Pathology

The alveolar walls are thickened and infiltrated with lymphocytes, plasma cells, and occasional eosinophils together with collections of histiocytes that, in some areas, form small granulomas. The small bronchioles are usually affected and there may be exudate in the lumen. Fibrotic changes occur in advanced cases.

Clinical Features

The disease occurs in either acute or chronic forms. In the former, symptoms of dyspnea, fever, shivering, and cough appear 4–6 hours after exposure and continue for 24–48 hours. The patient is frequently dyspneic at rest, with fine crepitations throughout both lung fields. The disease may also occur in a chronic form without prior acute attacks. These patients present with progressive dyspnea, usually over a period of years. In the acute form, the chest radiograph may be normal, but frequently a military nodular infiltrate is present. In the chronic form, fibrosis of the upper lobes is commonly seen.

Pulmonary Function

In well-developed disease, the typical restrictive pattern is seen. This includes reduced lung volumes, low compliance, hypoxemia that worsens on exercise, normal or low arterial Pco_2, and a reduced diffusing capacity. In the early stages, variable degrees of airway obstruction may be present.

Interstitial Disease Caused by Drugs, Poisons, and Radiation

Various drugs may cause an acute pulmonary reaction, which can proceed to interstitial fibrosis. These drugs include busulfan (used in the treatment of chronic myeloid leukemia), the antibiotic nitrofurantoin, the cardiac antiarrhythmic agent amiodarone, and the cytostatic drug bleomycin. Other antineoplastic drugs can also cause fibrosis. Oxygen in high concentrations causes acute toxic changes with subsequent interstitial fibrosis (Figs. 5.3 and 9.4). Ingestion of the weedkiller paraquat results in the rapid development of lethal interstitial fibrosis. Therapeutic radiation, which includes lung in the field, causes acute pneumonitis followed by fibrosis.

Collagen Diseases

Interstitial fibrosis with a typical restrictive pattern may be found in patients with systemic sclerosis (generalized scleroderma). Dyspnea is often severe and out of proportion to the changes in radiologic appearance or lung function. Other connective tissue diseases that may produce fibrosis include systemic lupus erythematosus and rheumatoid arthritis.

Lymphangitis Carcinomatosa

This refers to the spread of carcinoma tissue through pulmonary lymphatics and may complicate carcinomas, chiefly of the stomach or breast. Dyspnea is prominent, and the typical restrictive pattern of lung function may be seen.

Diseases of the Pleura

Pneumothorax

Air can enter the pleural space either from the lung or, less commonly, through the chest wall. The pressure in the intrapleural space is normally subatmospheric as a result of the elastic recoil forces of the lung and chest wall. When air enters the space, the lung collapses and the rib cage springs out. (See West JB. Respiratory physiology–the essentials, ed. 5. Baltimore: Williams & Wilkins, 1995: p. 101.) These changes are evident on a chest radiograph (Fig. 5.8), which shows partial or complete collapse of the lung, overexpansion of the rib cage and depression of the diaphragm on the affected side, and sometimes displacement of the mediastinum away from the pneumothorax. These changes are most

Figure 5.8.   Chest radiograph showing a large right-sided spontaneous pneumothorax. Note the small, collapsed right lung, depression of the right hemidiaphragm, and overexpansion of the rib cage on the right.

evident if the pneumothorax is large, particularly if a tension pneumothorax is present (see later text).

Spontaneous Pneumothorax

This most common form of pneumothorax is caused by the rupture of a small bleb on the surface of the lung near the apex. It typically occurs in tall young males and may be related to the high mechanical stresses that occur in the upper zone of the upright lung (Fig. 3.5). The presenting symptom is often sudden pain on one side accompanied by dyspnea. On auscultation, breath sounds are reduced on the affected side and the diagnosis is readily confirmed by a radiograph.

The pneumothorax gradually absorbs because the sum of the partial pressures in the venous blood is considerably less than atmospheric pressure. Recurrent attacks may need surgical treatment to promote adhesions between the two pleural surfaces.

Tension Pneumothorax

In a small proportion of spontaneous pneumothoraces, the communication between the lung and the pleural space functions as a check valve. As a consequence, air enters the space during inspiration but cannot escape during expiration. The result is a large pneumothorax in which the pressure may considerably exceed atmospheric pressure and thus interfere with venous return to the thorax.

This is a medical emergency and is recognized by increasing respiratory distress, tachycardia, and signs of mediastinal shift, such as tracheal deviation and movement of the apex beat. The radiograph is usually diagnostic. Treatment consists of relieving the pressure by inserting a tube through the chest wall. This tube is connected to an underwater seal that allows air to escape from the chest but not to enter it.

Pneumothorax Complicating Lung Disease

This occurs in a variety of conditions, including rupture of a bulla in COPD or a cyst in advanced fibrotic disease. It also sometimes occurs during mechanical ventilation with high airway pressures (see Chapter 10).

Pulmonary Function

As would be expected, a pneumothorax reduces the FEV_1 and FVC. In practice, pulmonary function tests are rarely helpful in the management of these patients because the radiograph is so informative.

Pleural Effusion

This refers to fluid rather than air in the pleural space. It is not a disease in its own right, but it frequently accompanies serious disease, and an explanation should always be sought.

The patient often reports dyspnea if the effusion is large and there may be pleuritic pain from the underlying disease. The chest signs are often informative and include reduced movement of the chest on the affected side, absence of breath sounds, and dullness to percussion. The radiograph is diagnostic.

Pleural effusions can be divided into exudates and transudates according to whether their protein content is high or low. In addition, the lactic dehydrogenase (LDH) tends to be higher in transudates. Exudates typically occur with malignancies and infections, whereas transudates complicate severe heart failure and other edematous states. It is often necessary to aspirate an effusion, but treatment should be directed at the underlying cause. Pulmonary function is impaired as in pneumothorax, but the measurements are not required in practice.

Variants of pleural effusion include empyema (pyothorax), hemothorax, and chylothorax, which refer to the presence of pus, blood, and lymph, respectively, in the pleural space.

Pleural Thickening

Occasionally, a long-standing pleural effusion results in a rigid, contracted fibrotic pleura that splints the lung and prevents its expansion. This can result in a severe restrictive type of functional impairment, particularly if the disease is bilateral. Surgical stripping may be necessary.

Diseases of the Chest Wall

Scoliosis

Bony deformity of the chest can cause restrictive disease. Scoliosis refers to lateral curvature of the spine and kyphosis to posterior curvature. Scoliosis is more serious, especially if the angulation is high in the vertebral column. It is frequently associated with a backward protuberance of the ribs, giving the appearance of an added kyphosis. In most cases, the cause is unknown, although the condition is occasionally caused by bony tuberculosis or neuromuscular disease.

The patient initially reports dyspnea on exertion; breathing tends to be rapid and shallow. Hypoxemia later develops, and eventually carbon dioxide retention and cor pulmonale may supervene. Bronchitis is common if the patient smokes.

Pulmonary function tests show a potentially significant reduction in all lung volumes. Airway resistance is nearly normal if related to lung volume. However, there is inequality of ventilation, partly because of airway closure in dependent regions. Parts of the lung are compressed and there are often areas of atelectasis.

The hypoxemia is caused by ventilation–perfusion inequality. In advanced disease, a reduced ventilatory response to CO_2 can often be demonstrated. This reduction reflects the increased work of breathing caused by deformity of the chest wall. Not only is the chest wall stiff, but also the respiratory muscles operate inefficiently. The pulmonary vascular bed is restricted, causing a rise in pulmonary artery pressure, which is exaggerated by the alveolar hypoxia. Venous congestion and peripheral edema may develop. The patient may succumb to an intercurrent pulmonary infection or respiratory failure.

Ankylosing Spondylitis

In this disease of unknown etiology, there is a gradual but relentless onset of immobility of the vertebral joints and fixation of the ribs. As a result, the movement of the chest wall is grossly reduced. There is a reduction of FVC and TLC, but the FEV/FVC percent and the airway resistance are normal. The compliance of the chest wall may fall and there is often some uneven ventilation, probably secondary to the reduced lung volume. The lung itself remains normal in nearly all cases, and diaphragmatic movement is preserved. Respiratory failure does not occur.

Neuromuscular Disorders

Diseases affecting the muscles of respiration or their nerve supply include poliomyelitis, Guillain-Barré syndrome, amyotrophic lateral sclerosis, myasthenia gravis, and muscular dystrophies (Fig. 2.4). All these diseases can lead to dyspnea and respiratory failure. The inability of the patient to take in a deep breath is reflected in a reduced FVC, TLC, inspiratory capacity, and FEV_1.

It should be remembered that the most important muscle of respiration is the diaphragm, and patients with progressive disease often do not report dyspnea until the diaphragm is involved. By then their ventilatory reserve may be severely compromised. The progress of the disease can be monitored by measuring the FVC and the blood gases. The maximal inspiratory and expiratory pressures that the patient can develop are also reduced. Assisted ventilation (Chapter 10) may become necessary.

6

Vascular Diseases

Pulmonary Edema

Pulmonary edema is an abnormal accumulation of fluid in the extravascular spaces and tissues of the lung. It is an important complication of a variety of heart and lung diseases and may be life-threatening.

Pathophysiology

Figure 5.1 reminds us that the pulmonary capillary is lined by endothelial cells and surrounded by an interstitial space. Often the interstitium is narrow on one side of the capillary, where it is formed by the fusion of the two basement membranes, while on the other side it is wider and contains collagen fibers. This latter region is particularly important for fluid exchange. Between the interstitial and alveolar spaces is the alveolar epithelium, composed predominantly of type 1 cells, and the superficial layer of surfactant (not shown in Fig. 5.1).

The capillary endothelium is highly permeable to water and to many solutes, including small molecules and ions. Proteins have a restricted movement across the endothelium. By contrast, the alveolar epithelium is much less permeable, and even small ions are largely prevented from crossing by passive diffusion. In addition, the epithelium actively pumps water from the alveolar to the interstitial space probably using a sodium, potassium, ATPase pump (31).

Hydrostatic forces tend to move fluid out of the capillary into the interstitial space, while osmotic forces tend to keep it in. The movement of fluid across the endothelium is governed by Starling's equation:

$$\dot{Q} = K[(P_c - P_i) - \sigma(\pi_c - \pi_i)] \qquad \text{(Eq. 6.1)}$$

where $\dot{Q}$ is the net flow out of the capillary, K is the filtration coefficient, P_c and P_i are the hydrostatic pressures in the capillary and interstitial space respectively, π_c and π_i are the corresponding colloid osmotic pressures, and σ is the reflection coefficient. The last variable indicates the effectiveness of the membrane in preventing (reflecting) the passage of the protein compared with that of water across the endothelium, and the coefficient is reduced in diseases that damage the cells and increase the permeability.

Although this equation is valuable conceptually, its practical use is limited. Of the four pressures, only one, the colloid osmotic pressure within the capillary, is known with any certainty. Its value is approximately 28 mm Hg. The capillary hydrostatic pressure is probably halfway between arterial and venous pressures but varies markedly from top to bottom of the upright lung. The colloid osmotic pressure of the interstitial fluid is not known but is approximately 20 mm Hg in lung lymph. However, there is some question whether this lymph has the same protein concentration as the interstitial fluid around the capillaries. The interstitial hydrostatic pressure is unknown and is thought by some physiologists to be substantially below atmospheric pressure. The value of σ in the pulmonary capillaries is approximately 0.7. It is probable that the net pressure from the Starling equilibrium is outward, causing a lymph flow of perhaps 20 ml/hr.

The fluid that leaves the capillaries moves within the interstitial space of the alveolar wall and tracks to the perivascular and peribronchial interstitium (Fig. 6.1). This tissue normally forms a thin sheath around the pulmonary arteries, veins, and bronchi and contains the lymphatics. The alveoli themselves are devoid of lymphatics, but once the fluid reaches the perivascular and peribronchial interstitium, some of it is carried in the lymphatics while some moves through the loose interstitial tissue. The lymphatics actively pump the lymph toward the bronchial and hilar nodes.

If excessive amounts of fluid leak from the capillaries, two factors tend to limit this flow. The first is a fall in the colloid osmotic pressure of the interstitial fluid as the protein is diluted as a result of the faster filtration of water compared with protein. However, this factor does not operate if the permeability of the capillary is greatly increased. The second is a rise in hydrostatic pressure in the interstitial space, which reduces the net filtration pressure. Both factors act in a direction to reduce fluid movement out of the capillaries.

Two stages in the formation of pulmonary edema are recognized (Fig. 6.1). The first is *interstitial edema*, which is characterized by engorgement of the perivascular and peribronchial interstitial tissue (cuffing) as shown in Fig. 6.2. Widened lymphatics can be seen, and lymph flow increases. In addition, some widening of the interstitium of the alveolar wall occurs. Pulmonary function is little affected at this stage and the condition is difficult to recognize, although some radiologic changes may be seen (see later text).

The second stage is *alveolar edema* (Fig. 6.3) (32). Here, fluid moves across into the alveoli, which are filled one by one. As a result of surface tension forces, the edematous alveoli shrink in size. Ventilation is prevented, and to the extent that the alveoli remain perfused, shunting of blood occurs and hypoxemia is

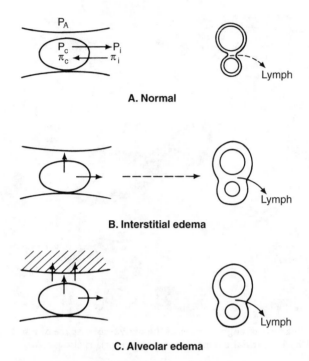

A. Normal

B. Interstitial edema

C. Alveolar edema

Figure 6.1. Stages of pulmonary edema. *(A)* There is normally a small lymph flow from the lung. *(B)* Interstitial edema. Here there is an increased flow with engorgement of the perivascular and peribronchial spaces and some widening of the alveolar wall interstitium. *(C)* Some fluid crosses the blood-gas barrier, producing alveolar edema.

inevitable. The edema fluid may move into the small and large airways and be coughed up as voluminous frothy sputum. In congestive heart failure, this sputum is pink because of the presence of red blood cells. What prompts the transition from interstitial to alveolar edema is not fully understood, but it may be that the lymphatics become overloaded and the pressure in the interstitial space increases so much that fluid spills over into the alveoli. Probably the alveolar epithelium is damaged and its permeability is increased. This would explain the presence of protein and red cells in the alveolar fluid.

Pathogenesis

This is best discussed under six headings, as shown in Table 6.1.

Increased Capillary Hydrostatic Pressure

This is the most common cause of pulmonary edema and frequently complicates heart disease, such as acute myocardial infarction, hypertensive left ventricular failure, and mitral valve disease. In all of these conditions, left atrial pressure rises, causing an increase in pulmonary venous and capillary pressures. This can be recognized at cardiac catheterization by measuring the "wedge" pressure (the

Figure 6.2.   Example of engorgement of the perivascular space of a small pulmonary blood vessel by interstitial edema. Some alveolar edema is also present.

Figure 6.3.   Section of dog lung showing alveolar edema. Note that some alveoli are filled completely while others are spared. The edematous alveoli tend to be smaller. (From Staub NC. The pathophysiology of pulmonary edema. Hum Pathol 1970;1:419–432.)

Table 6.1. Causes of Pulmonary Edema

Mechanism	Precipitating event
Increased capillary hydrostatic pressure	Myocardial infarction, mitral stenosis, fluid overload, pulmonary veno-occlusive disease
Increased capillary permeability	Inhaled or circulating toxins, sepsis, radiation oxygen toxicity, ARDS
Reduced lymph drainage	Increased central venous pressure, lymphangitis carcinomatosa
?Decreased interstitial pressure	Rapid removal of pleural effusion or pneumo-thorax, hyperinflation
Decreased colloid osmotic pressure	Overtransfusion hypoalbuminemia
Uncertain etiology	High altitude, neurogenic, overinflation, heroin

pressure in a catheter that has been wedged in a small pulmonary artery), which is approximately equal to pulmonary venous pressure.

Whether pulmonary edema occurs in these conditions depends on the rate of rise of the pressure. For example, in patients with mitral stenosis in whom the venous pressure is gradually raised over a period of years, remarkably high values may occur without clinical evidence of edema. This is partly because the caliber or number of the lymphatics increases to accommodate the higher lymph flow. However, these patients often have marked interstitial edema. By contrast, a patient with an acute myocardial infarction may develop alveolar edema with a smaller but more sudden rise in venous pressure.

Noncardiogenic causes also occur. Edema may be precipitated by excessive intravenous infusions of saline, plasma, or blood, leading to a rise in capillary pressure. Diseases of the pulmonary veins, such as pulmonary venoocclusive diseases, may also result in edema.

The cause of the edema in all these conditions is partly the increase in hydrostatic pressure, which disturbs the Starling equilibrium. However, recent work shows that when the pressure is raised to high levels, ultrastructural changes occur in the capillary walls, including disruption of the capillary endothelium, alveolar epithelium, or sometimes all layers of the wall. The result is an increase in permeability with movement of fluid, protein, and cells into the alveolar spaces. The condition is known as capillary stress failure (33).

One consequence is that for relatively small increases in pressure, the edema fluid has a low protein concentration because the permeability characteristics of the capillary wall are preserved (low-permeability edema). However, with large increases of pressure, the protein concentration of the edema fluid is high (high-permeability edema).

Increased Capillary Permeability

Apart from the situation referred to above, an increased capillary permeability also occurs in a variety of conditions. Toxins that are inhaled, such as chlorine, sulfur dioxide, or nitrogen oxides, or that circulate, such as alloxan or endotoxin, cause pulmonary edema in this way. Therapeutic radiation to the lung may cause edema and, ultimately, interstitial fibrosis. Oxygen poisoning produces a similar picture. Another cause is the adult respiratory distress syndrome (ARDS) (see Chapter 8). The edema fluid typically has a high protein concentration and contains many blood cells.

Reduced Lymph Drainage

This can be an exaggerating factor if another cause is present *Increased central venous pressure* may occur in ARDS, heart failure, and overtransfusion, and apparently interferes with the normal drainage of the thoracic duct. *Obstruction of lymphatics*, as in lymphangitis carcinomatosa, is another exaggerating cause.

Decreased Interstitial Pressure

This would be expected to promote edema from the Starling equation, although whether this occurs in practice is uncertain. However, patients who have a large unilateral pleural effusion or pneumothorax and a rapidly expanded lung sometimes develop pulmonary edema on that side. This may be partly related to the large mechanical forces acting on the interstitial space as the lung is expanded. However, the edema fluid is of the high-permeability type, and it is probable that the high mechanical stresses in the alveolar walls cause ultrastructural changes in the capillary walls (stress failure).

Decreased Colloid Osmotic Pressure

This is rarely responsible for pulmonary edema on its own, but it can exaggerate the edema that occurs when some other precipitating factor is present. Overtransfusion with saline is an important example; this has been implicated in the edema of the adult respiratory distress syndrome. Another example is the hypoproteinemia of the nephrotic syndrome.

Uncertain Etiology

This includes several forms of pulmonary edema. High altitude pulmonary edema occasionally affects climbers and skiers (Fig. 6.4). The wedge pressure is normal, so a raised pulmonary venous pressure is unlikely. However, the pulmonary artery pressure is high because of hypoxic vasoconstriction. One hypothesis is that the arteriolar constriction is uneven, and that regions of the capillary bed which are therefore not protected from the high pressure develop the ultrastructural changes of stress failure. This hypothesis would explain the high protein concentration in the alveolar fluid. Treatment is by descent to a lower altitude. Oxygen should be given if this is available.

Neurogenic pulmonary edema is seen after injuries to the central nervous system, for example, head trauma. The mechanism is probably stress failure of pulmonary capillaries after an acute rise in capillary pressure associated with heightened activity of the sympathetic nervous system.

Overinflation of the lung can cause pulmonary edema. This is sometimes seen

Figure 6.4.   Radiograph of a patient with pulmonary edema caused by high altitude.
Note the blotchy shadowing, especially on the right side.

in the intensive care unit when high levels of positive end-expiratory pressure (PEEP) are used (see Chapter 10). Again, the resulting large forces in the alveolar walls apparently damage the capillary walls.

Heroin overdosage can cause pulmonary edema. The complication is particularly seen in addicts who inject the drug intravenously when it is mixed with various diluents. These diluents might be partly responsible; however, edema can also follow oral ingestion.

Clinical Features

These features depend to some extent on the etiology of the edema, but some generalizations can be made. Dyspnea is usually a prominent symptom; breathing is typically rapid and shallow. Mild edema may cause few symptoms at rest, but exertional dyspnea is inevitable. Orthopnea (increased dyspnea while recumbent) is common. Paroxysmal nocturnal dyspnea (the patient awakes at night with severe dyspnea and wheezing) and Cheyne-Stokes respiration may occur. Cough is frequent and dry in the early stages. However, in fulminant edema, the patient may cough up large quantities of pink foamy sputum. Cyanosis may be present.

On auscultation, fine crepitations on inspiration are heard at the lung bases in early edema. In more severe cases, musical rhonchi may be heard. Abnormal heart sounds or murmurs are often present in cardiogenic edema.

Depending on the cause of the edema, the chest radiograph may show an enlarged heart and prominent pulmonary vessels. Interstitial edema causes septal lines to appear on the radiograph. These are short, linear, horizontal markings originating near the pleural surface in the lower zones that are caused by edematous interlobular septa. In more severe edema, blotchy shadowing occurs (Fig. 6.4). Occasionally, this shadow radiates from the hilar regions, giving a so-called bat's-wing or butterfly appearance. The explanation of this distribution is not clear but may be related to the perivascular and peribronchial cuffing that is particularly noticeable around the large vessels in the hilar region (Figs. 6.1 and 6.2).

Pulmonary Function

Extensive pulmonary function tests are seldom carried out on patients with pulmonary edema because they are so sick. The most important abnormalities are in the areas of mechanics and gas exchange.

Mechanics

Pulmonary edema reduces the distensibility of the lung and moves the pressure-volume curve downward and to the right (compare Fig. 3.1). An important factor in this is the alveolar flooding, which causes a reduction in volume of the affected lung units as a result of surface tension forces and reduces their participation in the pressure-volume curve. In addition, interstitial edema per se probably stiffens the lung by interfering with its elastic properties, although it is difficult to obtain clear evidence on this. Edematous lungs require abnormally large expanding pressures during mechanical ventilation and tend to collapse to abnormally small volumes when not actively inflated (Chapter 10).

Airway resistance is typically increased, especially if some of the larger airways contain edema fluid. Reflex bronchoconstriction after stimulation of irritant receptors in the bronchial walls may also play a role. It is possible that in the absence of alveolar edema, interstitial edema increases the resistance of small airways as a result of their peribronchial cuff (Fig. 6.1). This can be thought of as actually compressing the small airways or, at least, isolating them from the normal traction of the surrounding parenchyma (Fig. 6.5). There is some evidence that this mechanism increases the closing volume (Fig. 1.11) and thus predisposes to intermittent ventilation of dependent lung.

Gas Exchange

Interstitial edema has little effect on pulmonary gas exchange. A reduced diffusing capacity has sometimes been attributed to edematous thickening of the blood-

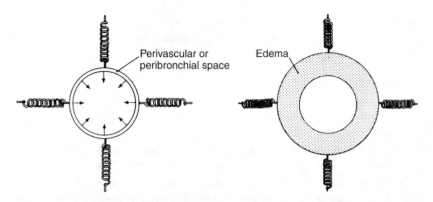

Figure 6.5.   Diagram showing how interstitial edema in the perivascular or peribron-chial region can reduce the caliber of the vessel or airway. The cuff isolates the structure from the traction of the surrounding parenchyma.

gas barrier, but the evidence is meager. It is possible that cuffs of interstitial edema around small airways (Figs. 6.1 and 6.5) can cause intermittent ventilation of dependent regions of the lung leading to hypoxemia, but the importance of this in practice is uncertain.

Alveolar edema causes hypoxemia chiefly because of blood flow to unventi-lated units (Fig. 10.4). These may be edema-filled alveoli or units supplied by airways that are completely obstructed by fluid. Hypoxic vasoconstriction tends to reduce the true shunt, but often this is large, as much as 50% or more of the total pulmonary blood flow in severe edema. Mechanical ventilation with positive end-expiratory pressure (PEEP) often substantially reduces the amount of shunt chiefly by clearing edema fluid from some of the larger airways (Fig. 10.4) although it may not reduce total lung water.

Lung units with low ventilation-perfusion ratios also contribute to the hypo-xemia. These presumably either lie behind airways partly obstructed by edema fluid or are units whose ventilation is reduced by their proximity to edematous alveoli. Such lung units are particularly liable to collapse during treatment with oxygen-enriched mixtures (Figs. 9.5 and 9.6), but oxygen therapy is often essen-tial to relieve the hypoxemia. A factor that often aggravates the hypoxemia caused by edema after acute myocardial infarction is a low cardiac output, which reduces the P_{O_2} in mixed venous blood.

The alveolar P_{CO_2} is often normal or low in pulmonary edema because of increased ventilation to the nonedematous alveoli. This is provoked in part by the arterial hypoxemia and also possibly by stimulation of lung receptors (see later text). However, in fulminating pulmonary edema, carbon dioxide retention and respiratory acidosis may develop.

Control of Ventilation

Patients with pulmonary edema typically have rapid, shallow breathing. This may be caused by stimulation of J receptors in the alveolar walls and perhaps other vagal afferents. The rapid breathing pattern minimizes the abnormally high elastic work of breathing. Arterial hypoxemia is an additional stimulus to breathing.

Pulmonary Circulation

Pulmonary vascular resistance rises, and hypoxic vasoconstriction of poorly ventilated or nonventilated areas is one mechanism for this. In addition, perivascular cuffing probably increases the resistance of the extra-alveolar vessels (Figs. 6.2 and 6.5). Other possible factors are the partial collapse of edematous alveoli, and alveolar wall edema that may compress or distort capillaries.

The topographical distribution of blood flow is sometimes altered by interstitial edema. The normal apex-to-base gradient becomes inverted, with the result that apical flow exceeds basal (Fig. 6.6). This is most commonly seen in patients with mitral stenosis. The cause is not fully understood, but it is possible that perivascular cuffs particularly increase the resistance of the lower zone vessels because the lung is less well expanded there (Fig. 3.5). This inverted distribution is not seen in noncardiogenic forms of edema, for example, ARDS.

Pulmonary Embolism

This important condition is often preventable and potentially fatal. Small emboli are common and are frequently undiagnosed.

Pathogenesis

Most pulmonary emboli arise as detached portions of venous thrombi that have formed in the deep veins of the lower extremities. Other sites include the right side of the heart and the pelvic area. Nonthrombotic emboli, such as fat, air, and amniotic fluid also occur but are relatively uncommon.

Figure 6.6.   Inversion of the topographic distribution of blood flow in a patient with mitral stenosis. The cause is not certain, but interstitial cuffs of edema around the lower zone vessels (Figures 6.2 and 6.5) may be partly responsible.

Factors that favor the formation of venous thrombi are:

1. Stasis of blood
2. Alterations in the blood coagulation system
3. Abnormalities of the vessel wall

Stasis of blood is promoted by immobilization following a fracture or an operation, local pressure, or venous obstruction. It is common in congestive heart failure, shock, hypovolemia, dehydration, and varicose veins. An enlarged fibrillating right atrium often contains thrombosed blood.

The intravascular *coagulability of blood* is increased in several conditions, such as polycythemia vera and sickle cell disease. The viscosity of the blood increases, thus favoring sluggish flow next to the vessel wall. In other conditions, the mechanism of increased coagulability is poorly understood. Such conditions include malignant diseases, pregnancy, recent trauma, and the use of oral contraceptives. There is no reliable test of an increased tendency for intravascular coagulation.

The *vessel wall may be damaged* by local trauma or by inflammation. Where there is marked local phlebitis with tenderness, redness, warmth, and swelling, the clot may be more securely adherent to the wall.

The presence of thrombosis in the deep veins of the legs or pelvis is often unsuspected until embolism occurs. Sometimes there is swelling of the limb or local tenderness, and there may be signs of inflammation. Acute dorsiflexion of the ankle may elicit calf pain. Ancillary tests, such as venography, the local uptake of radioactive fibrogen, and impedance plethysmography, may provide confirmation.

When the thrombus fragment is released, it is rapidly swept into one of the pulmonary arteries. Very large thrombi impact in a large artery. However, the thrombus may break up and block several smaller vessels. The lower lobes are frequently involved because they have a high blood flow (Fig. 3.5).

Pulmonary infarction, that is, death of the embolized tissue, occurs infrequently. More often there is distal hemorrhage and atelectasis, but the alveolar structures remain viable. Infarction is more likely if the embolus completely blocks a large artery or if there is preexisting lung or heart disease. Infarction results in alveolar filling with extravasated red cells and inflammatory cells and causes an opacity on the radiograph. Rarely, the infarct becomes infected, leading to an abscess. The infrequency of infarction can be explained, in part, by the fact that most emboli do not obstruct the vessel completely. In addition, bronchial artery anastomoses and the airways supply oxygen to the lung parenchyma.

Clinical Features

The presentation depends considerably on the size of the embolus and the patient's preexisting cardiopulmonary status.

Medium-Sized Emboli

These often present with pleuritic pain accompanied by dyspnea, slight fever, and cough productive of blood-streaked sputum. On auscultation, tachycardia is common and there may be a pleural friction rub. A small pleural effusion may develop. Embolism may mimic pneumonia, and recognition depends on being suspicious of the diagnosis. The chest radiograph is usually normal; a peripheral wedge-shaped shadow suggests infarction. A lung scan made after injecting radioactive albumin aggregates into the venous circulation shows one or more areas of reduced perfusion (Fig. 6.7). The distribution of ventilation, measured

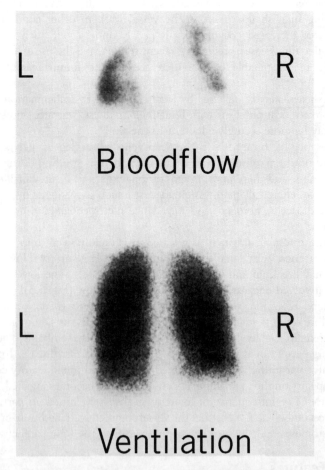

Figure 6.7.   Lung scan in a patient with multiple pulmonary emboli. The perfusion image (made with technetium-99m albumin) shows areas of absent blood flow in both lungs. The ventilation image (made with xenon-133) shows a normal pattern.

with radioactive gases or aerosols, is typically normal unless there is preexisting lung disease.

Massive Emboli

These may produce sudden hemodynamic collapse with shock, pallor, central chest pain, and sometimes loss of consciousness. The pulse is rapid and weak, the blood pressure is low, and the neck veins are engorged. The electrocardiogram may show the pattern of right ventricular strain. The prognosis is variable, but some 30% of massive emboli prove fatal.

Small Emboli

These are frequently unrecognized. However, repeated small emboli gradually oblate the pulmonary capillary bed, resulting in pulmonary hypertension. There is prominent dyspnea on exercise and this may lead to syncope. On examination, a right ventricular heave may be felt, and a loud pulmonary second sound may be heard. The ECG and chest radiograph confirm right ventricular hypertrophy.

Pulmonary Function

Pulmonary Circulation

This normally has a large reserve capacity because many capillaries are unfilled. When the pulmonary artery pressure rises, for example, on exercise, these capillaries are recruited and, in addition, some capillary distention occurs. This reserve means that at least half of the pulmonary circulation can be obstructed by an embolus before there is a substantial rise in pulmonary artery pressure.

In addition to the purely mechanical effects of the embolus, there is some evidence that active vasoconstriction occurs, at least for some minutes after embolization (Fig. 6.8). The mechanism is not understood, but in experimental animals, local release of serotonin from platelets associated with the embolus has been implicated, as well as reflex vasoconstriction via the sympathetic nervous system. It is not known to what extent these factors operate in humans.

If the embolus is large and if the pulmonary artery pressure rises considerably, the right ventricle may begin to fail. The end-diastolic pressure increases, arrhythmias may develop, and the tricuspid valve may become incompetent. In a few cases, pulmonary edema has been seen. This is presumably caused by leakage from those capillaries not protected from the raised pulmonary artery pressure (compare high altitude pulmonary edema).

The increase in pulmonary artery pressure gradually subsides over the subsequent days as the embolus resolves. This occurs both through fibrinolysis and also through organization of the clot into a small fibrous scar attached to the vessel wall. Patency of the vessel is thus usually restored.

Mechanics

When a pulmonary artery is occluded by a catheter in humans and experimental animals, the ventilation to that area of lung is reduced (34). The mechanism

Figure 6.8.   Transient changes in pulmonary artery pressure (related to cardiac out-put), arterial Po₂, and physiological dead space in dogs following experimental throm-boembolism. These suggest active responses of the pulmonary circulation and airways. The importance of these mechanisms in man is unknown. (From Dantzker DR, Wagner PD, Tornabene VW, Alzaraki NP, West JB. Gas exchange after pulmonary thromboembolization in dogs. Circ Res 1978L;42:92−103.)

appears to be a direct effect of the reduced alveolar P_{CO_2} on the smooth muscle of the local small airways, causing bronchoconstriction. It can be reversed by adding carbon dioxide to the inspired gas.

Although this airway response to vascular obstruction is generally much weaker than the corresponding vascular response to airway obstruction (hypoxic vasoconstriction), it serves a similar homeostatic role. The reduction in airflow to the unperfused lung reduces the amount of wasted ventilation and thus the physiologic dead space. This mechanism is apparently short-lived or ineffective after pulmonary thromboembolism in humans because most measurements of the distribution of ventilation with radioactive xenon made some hours after the episode show no defect in the embolized area. However, in experimental animals, transient changes in alveolar P_{O_2}, physiologic dead space, and airway resistance often occur after thromboembolism (Fig. 6.8) (35).

The elastic properties of the embolized region may change some hours after the event. In experimental animals, ligation of one pulmonary artery is followed by patchy hemorrhagic edema and atelectasis in the affected lung within 24 hours. This has been attributed to loss of pulmonary surfactant, which has a rapid turnover and apparently cannot be replenished in a lung that has lost its pulmonary blood flow. Again, it is not yet clear how often this occurs in human pulmonary thromboembolism or whether it is part of the pathological process that has been traditionally called infarction. The fact that most emboli do not completely block the vessel presumably limits its occurrence.

Gas Exchange

Moderate hypoxemia without carbon dioxide retention is often seen after pulmonary embolism. Both the physiologic shunt and dead space are increased. Various explanations for the hypoxemia have been advanced, including diffusion impairment in areas with high flows and therefore reduced transit time (Fig. 2.5), opening up of latent pulmonary artery-vein anastomoses as a consequence of the high pulmonary artery pressure, and blood flow through infarcted areas.

Measurements by the multiple inert gas elimination technique show that the hypoxemia can be explained by ventilation–perfusion inequality (36). Figure 6.9 shows distributions from two patients after massive pulmonary embolism. The most striking features are the large shunts (blood flow to unventilated alveoli) of 20% and 39% and the existence of lung units with high ventilation–perfusion ratios. The latter feature can be explained by the embolized regions where the blood flow is typically greatly reduced but not abolished completely. The precise mechanism of the shunts is not certain, but it may be blood flow through areas of hemorrhagic atelectasis.

Sometimes, patients with pulmonary embolism also show blood flow to poorly ventilated lung units. It is of interest that in experimental thromboembolism in dogs, no true shunt is typically seen, but the hypoxemia can be explained by the increased blood flow through the nonembolized areas of lung. This results in regions with low ventilation–perfusion ratios which depress the alveolar P_{O_2}. It is not clear how often this pattern occurs in human disease, but it is difficult to make many measurements in these patients because they are usually very ill.

The arterial P_{CO_2} after pulmonary embolism is maintained at the normal level by increasing the ventilation to the alveoli (Fig. 2.10). The increase in ventilation may be substantial because of the large physiologic dead space, and therefore wasted ventilation, caused by the embolized areas.

Some investigators have suggested that the difference in P_{CO_2} between arterial blood and end-tidal gas is a useful test for pulmonary embolism. The mixed alveolar P_{CO_2} tends to be low because of the high $\dot{V}_A/\dot{Q}$ in the embolized region, and because there is little uneven ventilation in this disease, the end-tidal P_{CO_2} is a useful measure of the mixed alveolar value.

In practice, this test is less sensitive than originally anticipated for two reasons. First, many emboli do not cause complete occlusion of the vessel, with the result that the P_{CO_2} in the affected region is not reduced to very low levels. Second, insofar as the embolized areas are poorly ventilated because of local bronchoconstriction, their contribution to end-tidal gas is reduced.

Figure 6.9.   **Distributions of ventilation-perfusion ratios in two patients with acute massive pulmonary embolism.** Note that in both instances, the hypoxemia could be explained by large shunts (blood flow to unventilated lung). In addition, there was a large increase in ventilation to lung units with abnormally high ventilation-perfusion ratios representing the embolized regions. (From D'Alonzo GE, Bower JS, DeHart P, and Dantzker DR. The mechanisms of abnormal gas exchange in acute massive pulmonary embolism. Am Rev Respir Dis 1983;128:170–172.)

Pulmonary Hypertension

The normal mean pulmonary artery pressure is approximately 15 mm Hg; an increased level is called pulmonary hypertension. Three principal mechanisms are listed.

1. *Increase in Left Atrial Pressure.* Examples are mitral stenosis or left ventricular failure. This is sometimes called passive pulmonary hypertension because the changes in pulmonary artery pressure are led by those in the left atrium. However, sustained increases in left atrial pressure lead to structural changes in the walls of the small pulmonary arteries, including medial hypertrophy and intimal thickening. Clinically, an increase in left atrial pressure can cause dyspnea, hemoptysis, and pulmonary edema.

2. *Increase in Pulmonary Blood Flow.* This occurs in congenital heart disease with left-to-right shunts through ventricular or atrial septal defects or a patent ductus arteriosus. Initially, the rise in pulmonary artery pressure is relatively small because of the ability of the pulmonary capillaries to accommodate high flows by recruitment and distension. However, sustained high flows result in structural changes in the walls of the small arteries, and eventually the pulmonary artery pressures may reach systemic levels, causing some right-to-left shunting and arterial hypoxemia.

3. *Increase in Pulmonary Vascular Resistance.* This is the most common cause of severe pulmonary hypertension. Again, three categories can be described:

   a. Vasoconstrictive, principally because of alveolar hypoxia as occurs at high altitude. This is also a component in the hypertension of chronic bronchitis and emphysema. Serotonin may cause transient vasoconstriction after thromboembolism, and the release of catecholamines may be a factor in some conditions, for example, neurogenic pulmonary edema. Other mediators have also been implicated, e.g., in asthma (Fig. 4.17).

   b. Obstructive, as in thromboembolism. In addition, the vessels may be occluded by circulating fat, air, amniotic fluid, or cancer cells. In schistosomiasis, the parasites lodge in small arteries causing a marked reaction.

   c. Obliterative, as in emphysema, in which the capillary bed is partly destroyed (Figs. 4.2 and 4.3). Various forms of arteritis can also occur, such as in polyarteritis nodosa. Rarely, the small veins are involved, as in pulmonary veno-occlusive disease.

Primary Pulmonary Hypertension

This is an uncommon disorder of unknown cause; some cases may be caused by unrecognized, repeated small emboli. The majority of patients are females in the age range of 20–40 years. Histologic examination of the lung shows an increase in smooth muscle in the small pulmonary arteries.

The chief symptom is dyspnea on exercise. Syncope may occur. Examination reveals signs of right ventricular hypertrophy that are confirmed by the ECG and chest radiographic appearances. Hypoxemia may be present, but ventilatory tests are usually normal. The disease typically progresses inexorably and death occurs within a few years. If the cause is repeated thromboembolism, surgery to remove the obstruction is sometimes valuable.

Cor Pulmonale

This term refers to right heart disease secondary to primary disease of the lung. The occurrence of right ventricular hypertrophy and fluid retention in COPD was discussed in Chapter 4. The same findings may occur late in restrictive lung disease.

The various factors that lead to pulmonary hypertension include obliteration of the capillary bed by destruction of alveolar walls or interstitial fibrosis, obstruction by thromboemboli, hypoxic vasoconstriction, hypertrophy of smooth muscle in the walls of the small arteries, and increased viscosity of the blood caused by polycythemia. Whether the term "right heart failure" should be applied to all these patients is disputed. In some, the output of the heart is increased because it is operating high on the Starling curve, and the output can increase further on exercise. The principal physiological abnormality in these patients is fluid retention. However, in others, true failure develops. Some physicians restrict the term cor pulmonale to those patients who have ECG evidence of right ventricular hypertrophy.

Pulmonary Arteriovenous Fistula

This uncommon condition is characterized by an abnormal communication between a pulmonary artery and vein. Approximately half of these patients also have telangiectases of the skin or mucous membranes, suggesting the presence of a general vascular defect. There is sometimes a family history of telangiectasia.

Small lesions cause no functional disturbances and may be found on a routine chest radiograph. Larger fistulae cause true shunts and hypoxemia. The arterial P_{O_2} is depressed far below the expected value during oxygen breathing (Fig. 2.7). Sometimes a bruit can be detected over the fistula by auscultation. Finger clubbing is common.

7

Environmental and Other Diseases

Diseases Caused By Inhaled Particles

Many occupational or industrial lung diseases are caused by inhaled dusts. Atmospheric pollutants are also important factors in the etiology of other diseases, such as chronic bronchitis, emphysema, asthma, and bronchial carcinoma, so we shall start by looking at the environment in which we all live.

Atmospheric Pollutants

Carbon Monoxide

This is the largest pollutant by weight in the United States (Fig. 7.1, *left*). It is produced by the incomplete combustion of carbon in fuels, chiefly in the automobile engine (Fig. 7.1, *right*). The main hazard of carbon monoxide is its propensity to tie up hemoglobin; because carbon monoxide has over 200 times the affinity of oxygen, it competes successfully with this gas. (See West JB. Respiratory physiology–the essentials, ed. 5. Baltimore: Williams & Wilkins, 1995: p. 76.) A commuter using a busy urban freeway may have 5–10% of his or her hemoglobin bound to carbon monoxide, particularly if he or she is a cigarette smoker. There is evidence that this can impair mental skills. The emission of carbon monoxide and other pollutants by automobile engines can be reduced by installing a catalytic converter that processes the exhaust gases.

Nitrogen Oxides

These are produced when fossil fuels (coal, oil) are burned at high temperatures in power stations and automobiles. These gases cause inflammation of the eyes

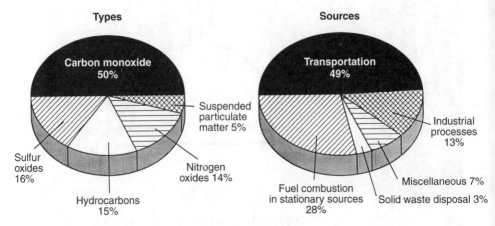

Figure 7.1.   Air pollutants (by weight) in the United States. Note that transportation sources, especially automobiles, account for the largest amount of pollutants. Stationary sources, particularly power stations, account for 28%. (From the Environmental Protection Agency.)

and upper respiratory tract during smoggy conditions. At higher concentrations, they can cause acute tracheitis, acute bronchitis, and pulmonary edema. The yellow haze of smog is a result of these gases.

Sulfur Oxides

These are corrosive, poisonous gases produced when sulfur-containing fuels are burned, chiefly by power stations. These gases cause inflammation of the mucous membranes, eyes, upper respiratory tract, and bronchial mucosa. Short-term exposure to high concentrations causes pulmonary edema. Long-term exposure to lower levels results in chronic bronchitis in experimental animals. The best way to reduce emissions of sulfur oxides is to use low-sulfur fuels, but these are more expensive.

Hydrocarbons

Hydrocarbons, like carbon monoxide, represent unburned wasted fuel. They are not toxic at concentrations normally found in the atmosphere. However, they are hazardous because they form photochemical oxidants under the influence of sunlight (see later text).

Particulate Matter

This includes particles with a wide range of sizes, up to visible smoke and soot. Major sources are power stations and industrial plants. Often their emission can be reduced by processing the waste air stream by filtering or scrubbing, although removing the smallest particles is often expensive.

Photochemical Oxidants

These include ozone and other substances, such as peroxyacyl nitrates, aldehydes, and acrolein. They are not primary emissions but are produced by the action of sunlight on hydrocarbons and nitrogen oxides. They cause inflammation of the eyes and respiratory tract, damage to vegetation, and offensive odors. In higher concentrations, ozone causes pulmonary edema. These oxidants contribute to the thick haze of smog.

The concentration of atmospheric pollutants is often greatly increased by a temperature inversion, that is, a low layer of cold air beneath warmer air. This prevents the normal escape of warm surface air with its pollutants to the upper atmosphere. The deleterious effects of a temperature inversion are particularly marked in a low lying area surrounded by hills, such as the Los Angeles basin.

Cigarette Smoke

This is one of the most important pollutants in practice because it is inhaled by devotees in concentrations many times greater than are pollutants in the atmosphere. It includes approximately 4% carbon monoxide, enough to raise the carboxyhemoglobin level in a smoker's blood to 10%. This percentage is sufficient to impair exercise and mental performance. The smoke also contains the alkaloid nicotine which stimulates the autonomic nervous system, causing tachycardia, hypertension, and sweating. Aromatic hydrocarbons and other sub-stances, loosely called "tars," are apparently responsible for the high risk of bronchial carcinoma in cigarette smokers. A male who smokes 35 cigarettes/day has 40 times the risk of a nonsmoker. Increased risks of chronic bronchitis and emphysema and of coronary heart disease are also well documented. A single cigarette causes a marked increase in airway resistance in many smokers and nonsmokers (Fig. 3.2).

Deposition of Aerosols in the Lung

The term "aerosol" refers to a collection of particles that remains airborne for a substantial amount of time. Many pollutants exist in this form, and their pattern of deposition in the lung depends chiefly on their size. The properties of aerosols are also important in understanding the fate of inhaled bronchodila-tors. Three mechanisms of deposition are recognized (37).

Impaction

Impaction refers to the tendency of the largest inspired particles to fail to turn the corners of the respiratory tract. As a result, many particles impinge on the mucous surfaces of the nose and pharynx (Fig. 7.2A) and also on the bifurcations of the large airways. Once a particle strikes a wet surface, it is trapped and not subsequently released. The nose is remarkably efficient at removing the largest particles by this mechanism; almost all particles greater than 20 μm in diameter and approximately 95% of particles 5 μm in diameter are filtered by the nose during resting breathing. Figure 7.3 shows that most of the deposition of particles over 3 μm in diameter occurs in the nasopharynx during nose breathing.

Sedimentation

Sedimentation is the gradual settling of particles because of their weight (Fig. 7.2B). It is particularly important for medium-sized particles (1–5 μm) because

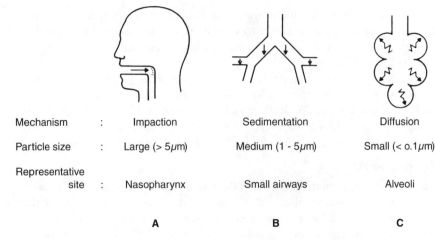

Mechanism	:	Impaction	Sedimentation	Diffusion
Particle size	:	Large (> 5μm)	Medium (1 - 5μm)	Small (< o.1μm)
Representative site	:	Nasopharynx	Small airways	Alveoli

	A	B	C

Figure 7.2.   Scheme of deposition of aerosols in the lung. The term "representative sites" does not mean that these are the only sites where this form of deposition occurs. For example, impaction also occurs in the medium-sized bronchi, and diffusion also occurs in the large and small airways. (See text for details.)

the larger particles are removed by impaction and the smaller particles settle so slowly. Deposition by sedimentation occurs extensively in the small airways, including the terminal and respiratory bronchioles. The chief reason is simply that the dimensions of those airways are small and therefore the particles have a shorter distance to fall. Note that the particles, unlike gases, are not able to diffuse from the respiratory bronchioles to the alveoli because of their negligibly small diffusion rate. (See West JB. Respiratory physiology–the essentials, ed. 5. Baltimore: Williams & Wilkins, 1995: p. 6.)

Figure 7.4 shows accumulations of dust around the terminal and respiratory bronchioles of a coal miner with early pneumoconiosis (38). Although the retention of dust depends on both deposition and clearance, and it is likely that some of this dust was transported from peripheral alveoli, the appearance is a graphic reminder of the vulnerability of this region of the lung. It has been suggested that some of the earliest changes in chronic bronchitis and emphysema are secondary to the deposition of atmospheric pollutants (including tobacco smoke particles) in these small airways.

Diffusion

Diffusion is the random movement of particles as a result of their continuous bombardment by gas molecules (Fig. 7.2C). It occurs to a significant extent only in the smallest particles less than 0.1 μm in diameter. Deposition by diffusion chiefly takes place in the small airways and alveoli where the distances to the

Figure 7.3. Site of deposition of aerosols. Note that the largest particles remain the nasopharynx, but the small particles can penetrate to the alveoli.

wall are least. However, some deposition by this mechanism also occurs in the larger airways.

Many inhaled particles are not deposited at all but are exhaled with the next breath. In fact, only some 30% of 0.5 μm particles may be left in the lung during normal resting breathing. These particles are too small to impact or sediment to a large extent. In addition, they are too large to diffuse significantly. As a result, they do not move from the terminal and respiratory bronchioles to the alveoli by diffusion, which is the normal mode of gas movement in this region. Small particles may become larger during inspiration by aggregation or by absorbing water.

The pattern of ventilation affects the amount of aerosol deposition. Slow, deep breaths increase the penetration into the lung and thus increase the amount of dust deposited by sedimentation and diffusion. Exercise results in higher rates of airflow and it particularly increases deposition by impaction. In general, deposition of dust is proportional to the ventilation during exercise, which is therefore an important factor during work at the coal face, for example.

Clearance of Deposited Particles

Fortunately, the lung is efficient at removing particles that are deposited within it. Two distinct clearance mechanisms exist: the mucociliary system and the alveolar macrophages (Fig. 7.5).

Figure 7.4.   Section of lung from a coal miner showing accumulations of dust around the respiratory bronchioles. These small airways show some dilatation, sometimes called focal emphysema. (From Heppleston AG, Leopold JG. Chronic pulmonary emphysema: anatomy and pathogenesis. Am J Med 1961;31:279–291.)

Mucociliary System

Mucus is produced by two sources: 1) Bronchial seromucous glands situated deep in the bronchial walls (Figs. 4.6, 4.7, and 7.6). Both mucus-producing and serous-producing cells are present, and ducts lead the mucus to the airway surface. 2) Goblet cells, which form part of the bronchial epithelium.

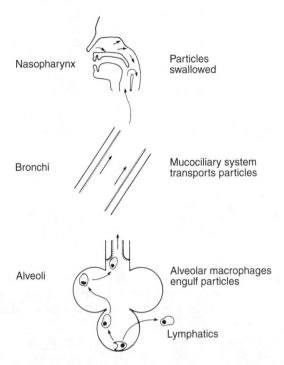

Figure 7.5. Clearance of inhaled particles from the lung. Particles that deposit on the surface of the airways are transported by the mucociliary escalator and swallowed. Particles that reach the alveoli are engulfed by macrophages, which either migrate to the ciliary surface or escape via the lymphatics.

The normal mucous film is approximately 5–10 μm thick and has two layers (Fig. 7.6). The superficial gel layer is relatively tenacious and viscous. As a result, it is efficient at trapping deposited particles. The deeper sol layer is less viscous and thus allows the cilia to beat within it easily. It is likely that the abnormal retention of secretions that occurs in some diseases is caused by changes in the composition of the mucus, with the result that it cannot be easily propelled by the cilia.

The mucus contains the immunoglobulin IgA, which is derived from plasma cells and lymphoid tissue. This humoral factor is an important defense against foreign proteins, bacteria, and viruses.

The cilia are 5–7 μm in length and beat in a synchronized fashion at between 1000 and 1500 times/min. During the forward stroke, the tips of the cilia apparently come in contact with the gel layer, thus propelling it. However, during the recovery phase, the cilia are bent so much that they move entirely within the sol layer where the resistance is less.

The mucous blanket moves up at about 1 mm/min in small peripheral airways but as fast as 2 cm/min in the trachea, and eventually the particles reach the

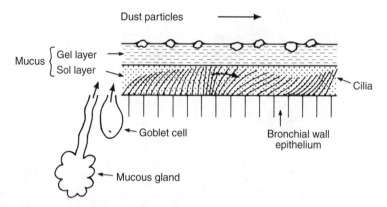

Figure 7.6.   Mucociliary escalator. The mucous film consists of a superficial gel layer that traps inhaled particles and a deeper sol layer. It is propelled by cilia.

level of the pharynx where they are swallowed. The clearance of a healthy bronchial mucosa is essentially complete in less than 24 hours. In very dusty environments, mucous secretion may be increased so much that cough and expectoration assist in the clearance.

The normal operation of the mucociliary system is affected by pollution or disease. The cilia apparently can be paralyzed by the inhalation of toxic gases, such as oxides of sulfur and nitrogen and perhaps by tobacco smoke. In acute inflammation of the respiratory tract, the bronchial epithelium may be denuded. Changes in the character of the mucus may occur with infection, thus making it difficult for the cilia to transport it. Mucous plugging of bronchi occurs in asthma, but the mechanism is unknown. Finally, in chronic infections such as bronchiectasis or chronic bronchitis, the volume of secretions may be so great that the ciliary transport system is overloaded.

Alveolar Macrophages

The mucociliary system stops short of the alveoli, and particles deposited there are engulfed by macrophages. These amoeboid cells roam around the surface of the alveoli. When they phagocytose foreign particles, they either migrate to the small airways where they load on to the mucociliary escalator (Fig. 7.5) or they leave the lung in the lymphatics or possibly the blood. When the dust burden is large or the dust particles are toxic, some of the macrophages migrate through the walls of the respiratory bronchioles and dump their dust there. Figure 7.4 shows accumulations of dust around the respiratory bronchioles in the lung of a coal miner (38). If the dust is toxic, such as silica, a fibrous reaction is stimulated in this region.

The macrophages not only transport bacteria out of the lung but also kill them in situ by means of the lysozymes they contain. As a consequence, the alveoli quickly become sterile, although it takes some time for the dead organisms to be cleared from the lung. Immunologic mechanisms are also important in the antibacterial action of macrophages.

Normal macrophage activity can be impaired by various factors, such as cigarette smoke, oxidant gases such as ozone, alveolar hypoxia, radiation, the administration of corticosteroids, and the ingestion of alcohol. Macrophages that engulf particles of silica are often destroyed by this toxic material.

Coal Workers' Pneumoconiosis

The term "pneumoconiosis" refers to parenchymal lung disease caused by inorganic dust inhalation. One form is seen in coal workers and it is directly related to the amount of coal dust to which the miner has been exposed.

Pathology

Early and late forms of the disease should be distinguished. In simple pneumoconiosis, there are aggregations of coal particles around terminal and respiratory bronchioles, with some dilatation of these small airways (Fig. 7.4). In the advanced form of the disease, known as progressive massive fibrosis, condensed masses of black fibrous tissue infiltrated with dust are seen. Only a small fraction of miners exposed to heavy dust concentrations develop progressive massive fibrosis.

Clinical Features

Simple pneumoconiosis apparently causes little disability despite its radiographic appearances. The dyspnea and cough that often accompany the disease are closely related to the smoking history of the miner and are probably chiefly caused by associated chronic bronchitis and emphysema. By contrast, progressive massive fibrosis usually causes increasing dyspnea and may terminate in respiratory failure.

The chest radiograph of simple pneumoconiosis shows a delicate micronodular mottling, and various stages in the advance of the disease are recognized depending on the density of the shadows. Progressive massive fibrosis results in large, irregular dense opacities often surrounded by abnormally radiolucent lung. Figure 7.7 shows an unusual example in which simple pulmonary function tests were within normal limits despite the striking amount of lung disease (39).

Pulmonary Function

Simple pneumoconiosis usually causes little functional impairment by itself. However, sometimes a small reduction in forced expiratory volume, a rise in residual volume, and a fall in arterial Po_2 are seen. It is often difficult to know whether these changes are caused by associated chronic bronchitis and emphysema.

Progressive massive fibrosis causes a mixed obstructive and restrictive pattern. Distortion of the airways results in irreversible obstructive changes, whereas the large masses of fibrous tissue reduce the useful volume of the lung. Increasing hypoxemia, cor pulmonale, and terminal respiratory failure may occur.

Silicosis

This pneumoconiosis is caused by the inhalation of silica (SiO_2) during quarrying, mining, or sandblasting. Whereas coal dust is virtually inert, silica particles are toxic and provoke a severe fibrous reaction in the lung.

Figure 7.7.   Chest radiograph of an 81-year-old coal miner with advanced bilateral progressive massive fibrosis. Astonishingly, simple pulmonary function tests were within normal limits for his age. For example, his arterial Po_2 and Pco_2 were 79 and 36 mm Hg, respectively. (From Ulmer WT, Reichel G. Functional impairment in coal worker's pneumoconiosis. Ann N Y Acad Sci 1972;200:405–412.)

Pathology

Silicotic nodules composed of concentric whorls of dense collagen fibers are found around respiratory bronchioles, inside alveoli, and along the lymphatics. Silica particles may be seen in the nodules.

Clinical Features

Mild forms of the disease may cause no symptoms, although the chest radiograph shows fine nodular markings. Advanced disease results in cough and severe dyspnea, especially on exercise. The radiograph sometimes shows streaks of fibrous tissue, and progressive massive fibrosis may develop. The disease may progress long after exposure to the dust has ceased. There is an increased risk of pulmonary tuberculosis.

Pulmonary Function

The changes are similar to those seen in coal workers' pneumoconiosis but are often more severe. In advanced disease, generalized interstitial fibrosis may develop, with a restrictive type of defect, severe dyspnea and hypoxemia on exercise, and a reduced diffusing capacity.

Asbestos-related Diseases

Asbestos is a naturally occurring fibrous mineral silicate that is used in a variety of industrial applications, including heat insulation, pipe lagging, roofing materials, and brake linings. Asbestos fibers are long and thin, and it is possible that their aerodynamic characteristics allow them to penetrate far into the lung. When they are in the lung, they may become encased in proteinaceous material. If these are coughed up in the sputum, they are known as asbestos bodies.

Three health hazards are recognized:

1. Diffuse interstitial fibrosis (asbestosis) may gradually occur after heavy exposure. There is a progressive dyspnea (especially on exercise), weakness, and finger clubbing. On auscultation, there are fine basal crepitations. The chest radiograph shows haziness or mottling. Pulmonary function tests in advanced disease reveal a typical restrictive pattern with reductions of vital capacity and lung compliance. A fall in diffusing capacity occurs relatively early in the disease.
2. Bronchial carcinoma is a common complication. Cigarette smoking is often an aggravating factor.
3. Pleural disease may occur after trivial exposure, for example, in a person who washes the clothes of an asbestos worker. Pleural thickening and plaques are common but are usually harmless. Malignant mesothelioma may develop as much as 40 years after light exposure. It causes progressive restriction of chest movement, severe chest pain, and a rapid downhill course.

Other Pneumoconioses

A variety of other dusts cause simple pneumoconiosis. Examples include iron and its oxides, which cause siderosis and result in a striking, mottled radiographic appearance. Antimony and tin are other culprits. Beryllium exposure results in granulomatous lesions of acute or chronic types. The latter results in interstitial fibrosis with its typical restrictive pattern of dysfunction. The disease is now much less common than it was as a result of strict control of beryllium in industry.

Byssinosis

Some inhaled organic dusts cause airway reactions rather than alveolar reactions. A good example is byssinosis, which follows exposure to cotton dust, especially in the cardroom where the fibers are initially processed.

The pathogenesis is not fully understood, but it appears that the inhalation of some active component in the bracts (leaves around the stem of the cotton boll) leads to the release of histamine from mast cells in the lung. The resulting bronchoconstriction causes dyspnea and wheezing. A feature of the disease is that the symptoms are worse on entering the mill, especially after a period of absence. For this reason it is sometimes known as "Monday fever." The symptoms include dyspnea, tightness of the chest, wheezing, and an irritating cough. Workers who have already had chronic bronchitis or asthma are especially susceptible.

Pulmonary function tests show an obstructive pattern with reductions in FEV_1, FEV/FVC%, $FEF_{25-75\%}$, and FVC. Airway resistance measured in a body plethysmograph is increased. In addition, the amount of inequality of ventilation as determined by nitrogen washout rises after exposure. Typically, these abnormalities gradually become worse over the course of the working day, but partial or complete recovery occurs during the night or over the weekend. There is no evidence of parenchymal involvement, and the chest radiograph is normal. However, epidemiological studies show that daily exposure over 20 years or so causes permanent impairment of lung function of the type associated with COPD.

Occupational Asthma

Various occupations involve exposure to allergenic organic dusts, and some individuals develop hypersensitivity. These individuals include flour mill workers who are sensitive to the wheat weevil, printers exposed to gum acacia, and workers handling fur or feathers. Toluene diisocyanate (TDI) is a special case because some individuals develop an extreme sensitivity to this substance, which is used in the manufacture of polyurethane products.

Malignant Diseases

Bronchial Carcinoma

This important disease is only briefly discussed here because its effects on pulmonary function are minor in the context of diagnosis, staging, and treatment. The incidence of the disease is awesome; it is the most common form of malignancy in the male and accounts for 25% of all male cancer deaths. Much of this disease is preventable.

Etiology

There is overwhelming evidence that cigarette smoking is a major factor. Epidemiologic studies show that an individual who smokes 20 cigarettes a day has about 20 times the chance of dying from the disease compared with a nonsmoker of the same age and sex. Furthermore, the risk decreases dramatically if the individual stops smoking.

The specific causative agents in cigarette smoke are uncertain, but many potential carcinogenic substances are present, including aromatic hydrocarbons, phenols, and radioisotopes. Many smoke particles are submicronic and penetrate far into the lung. However, the fact that many bronchogenic carcinomas originate in the large bronchi suggests that deposition by impaction or sedimentation may play an important role (Fig. 7.2). Also, the large bronchi are exposed to a high concentration of tobacco smoke products as the material is transported from the more peripheral regions by the mucociliary system. Individuals who inhale other peoples' smoke (passive smokers) in an indoor area have an increased risk.

Other etiological factors are recognized. Urban dwellers are more at risk, suggesting that atmospheric pollution plays a part. This finding is hardly surprising in view of the variety of chronic respiratory tract irritants that exist in city air (Fig. 7.1). Occupational factors also exist, especially exposure to chromates, nickel, arsenic, asbestos, and radioactive gases.

Pathology

1. *Squamous carcinomas* are the most common cell type, accounting for nearly half of all cases. Microscopically, intercellular bridges are visible, keratin is present, and the cells often form a whorl or nest pattern. Cavitation sometimes occurs. There is often an initial response to radiation, but not to chemotherapy.

2. *Small cell carcinomas* contain a homogeneous population of oat-like cells giving a characteristic appearance. Up to one-third of all tumors are of this type; they are highly malignant with rapid dissemination. These tumors are seldom seen in peripheral lung and usually do not cavitate.

3. *Large cell undifferentiated carcinomas* contain cells of approximately the same size as squamous carcinomas, but the characteristic whorls are not seen. They tend to occur in the periphery of the lung. Approximately 10% of tumors are in this category.

4. *Adenocarcinomas* show glandular differentiation and often produce mucus. They typically occur peripherally, and the incidence of occurrence appears to be increasing and is greater in women.

5. *Alveolar cell carcinomas* arise from type II alveolar cells and are rare. They are not related to smoking. Some authorities regard these as a subset of adenocarcinomas.

Many tumors show some heterogeneity of cell type, thus making classification difficult.

Clinical Features

An unproductive cough or hemoptysis is a common early symptom. Sometimes hoarseness is the first clue and is caused by involvement of the left recurrent laryngeal nerve. Dyspnea caused by pleural effusion or bronchial obstruction, and chest pain caused by pleural involvement, usually are late symptoms. Examination of the chest is often negative, although signs of lobar collapse or consolidation may be found. The chest radiograph is often crucial, but a small carcinoma may not be visible. Bronchoscopy and sputum cytology are valuable aids to early diagnosis.

Pulmonary Function

The physician's objective is to diagnose a carcinoma of the bronchus early enough to remove it surgically. Pulmonary function tests are rarely of value in this regard. However, lung function is often impaired in moderately advanced disease.

A large pleural effusion causes a restrictive defect, as may the collapse of a lobe after complete bronchial obstruction. Partial obstruction of a large bronchus can result in an obstructive pattern. The obstruction can be caused either by a tumor of the bronchial wall or by compression by an enlarged lymph gland. Sometimes the movement of the lung on the affected side is seen to lag behind the normal lung, and air may cycle back and forth between the normal and obstructed lobes (see West JB. Respiratory physiology–the essentials, ed. 5. Baltimore: Williams & Wilkins, 1995: p. 161). This cycle is known as pendelluft (swinging air). Complete obstruction of a main stem bronchus can give a pseudo-restrictive pattern because half the lung is not ventilating. Partial or complete bronchial obstruction usually causes some hypoxemia.

Infectious Diseases

Although infectious diseases are of great importance in the general context of internal medicine, they do not generally cause specific patterns of impaired function, and pulmonary function tests are of little value in the management of patients with these diseases. This section is therefore brief.

Pneumonia

This term refers to inflammation of the lung parenchyma associated with alveolar filling by exudate.

Pathology

The alveoli are crammed with cells, chiefly polymorphonuclear leukocytes. Resolution often occurs with restoration of the normal morphology. However, suppuration may result in necrosis of tissue causing a lung abscess. Special forms of pneumonia include that following aspiration of gastric fluid or animal or mineral oil (lipoid pneumonia). Psittacosis is a form transmitted from infected parrots by a rickettsia.

Clinical Features

These features vary considerably depending on the causative organism, the age of the patient, and his or her general condition. The usual features include malaise, fever, and cough. Pleuritic pain is common and is worse on deep breathing. Examination reveals rapid shallow breathing, tachycardia, and sometimes cyanosis. There often are signs of consolidation, and the chest radiograph shows opacification. This may involve all of a lobe (lobar pneumonia), but frequently the distribution is patchy (bronchopneumonia). Sputum examination and culture frequently identify the causative organism.

Pulmonary Function

Because the pneumonic region is not ventilated, it causes shunting and hypoxemia. The severity of these conditions depend on the local pulmonary blood flow, which may be substantially reduced either by the disease process itself or by hypoxic vasoconstriction. However, patients with severe pneumonia may be cyanosed. Carbon dioxide retention does not generally occur. Chest movement may be restricted by pleural pain or by a pleural effusion.

Tuberculosis

Pulmonary tuberculosis takes many forms. Early lesions do not affect pulmonary function, but in the late stages of the disease, severe functional impairment may occur, leading to respiratory failure. Advanced disease is much less common now because of treatment with antituberculous drugs.

The initial infection results in a primary complex with hilar lymph node enlargement. This enlargement rapidly resolves and is usually not recognized. The postprimary infection is usually in the apices of the lungs, apparently because the high ventilation-perfusion ratio there and the resulting high P_{O_2} (Fig. 3.5) provide a favorable environment for the growth of the bacillus. If this infection heals, as it generally does, no functional impairment results.

Extension of the infection may cause pneumonia, miliary infection, cavitation, lobar collapse, or pleural effusion. Ultimately, severe fibrosis may develop, with restrictive impairment of function.

Pulmonary Involvement in AIDS

Acquired immunodeficiency syndrome (AIDS) frequently involves the lung. The most common infection is *Pneumocystis carinii*, but *Mycobacterium avium-intracellulare* and cytomegalovirus infections also occur often. Less frequent infections include tuberculosis and *Legionella*. Kaposi's sarcoma may occur in the lung. In patients from high-risk groups who present with these pulmonary problems, AIDS should be suspected.

Suppurative Diseases

Bronchiectasis

This disease is characterized by dilatation of bronchi with local suppuration.

Pathology

The mucosal surface of the affected bronchi shows loss of ciliated epithelium, squamous metaplasia, and infiltration with inflammatory cells. Pus is present in the lumen during infective exacerbations. The surrounding lung often shows fibrosis and old inflammatory changes.

Clinical Features

The disease usually follows childhood pneumonia, and the prevalence has fallen greatly since the introduction of powerful antibiotics. The cardinal feature is a productive cough with yellow or green sputum. This sputum may occur only after a cold or it may be present continuously. There may be hemoptysis and halitosis. Crepitations are often heard, and finger clubbing is seen in severe cases. The chest radiograph shows increased markings.

Pulmonary Function

Mild disease causes no loss of function. In more advanced cases, there is a reduction of FEV and FVC because of chronic inflammatory changes, including fibrosis. Radioactive gas measurements show reduced ventilation and pulmonary blood flow in the affected area, but there may be a greatly increased bronchial artery supply to the diseased tissue. Hypoxemia may develop as a result of blood flow through unventilated lung.

Cystic Fibrosis

This is a disease of all exocrine glands caused by a genetic abnormality affecting chloride and sodium transport. In the lung, it takes the form of bronchiectasis and bronchiolitis. Identification of the specific genetic defect has raised the possibility of effective gene therapy.

Pathology

The principal organ affected is the pancreas, where the tissue atrophies and the ducts remain as dilated cysts. The bronchiectasis results in part from excessive secretions from the hypertrophied mucous glands. Ciliary activity is also apparently impaired, and mucous plugging of small airways and chronic infection follow. Malnutrition secondary to pancreatic failure may lower resistance to infection.

Clinical Features

A few patients die of meconium ileus shortly after birth, and others remain small and malnourished. The respiratory symptoms include productive cough, frequent chest infections, and decreased exercise tolerance. Finger clubbing is often prominent. Auscultation may reveal coarse rales and rhonchi. The chest radiograph is abnormal early in the disease and shows areas of consolidation, fibrosis, and cystic changes. In young children, the finding of high sodium concentration in the sweat confirms the diagnosis.

Until recently, death almost invariably occurred before adulthood among patients with cystic fibrosis, but with improved treatment of chest infections, survival into the 20s is now sometimes seen. Indeed, the disease should be considered when a teenager or a young adult presents with features of chronic bronchitis.

Pulmonary Function

An abnormal distribution of ventilation and an increased alveolar–arterial O_2 difference are early changes. Some investigators report that tests of small airways function, such as flow rates at low lung volumes, may detect minimal disease. There is a decrease in FEV_1 and $FEF_{25-75\%}$ that does not respond to bronchodilators. RV and FRC are raised and there may be loss of elastic recoil. Exercise tolerance falls as the disease progresses.

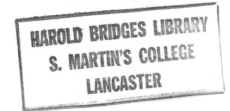
HAROLD BRIDGES LIBRARY
S. MARTIN'S COLLEGE
LANCASTER

Part
Three

Function of the Failing Lung

8. Respiratory Failure
9. Oxygen Therapy
10. Mechanical Ventilation

Respiratory failure is the end result of many types of acute or chronic lung disease. Part Three is devoted to the physiological principles of respiratory failure and its chief modes of treatment: oxygen administration and mechanical ventilation.

8

Respiratory Failure

Respiratory failure is said to occur when the lung fails to oxygenate the arterial blood adequately and/or fails to prevent CO_2 retention. There is no absolute definition of the levels of arterial PO_2 and PCO_2 that indicate respiratory failure. However, a PO_2 of less than 60 mm Hg or a PCO_2 of more than 50 mm Hg are numbers that are often quoted. In practice, the significance of such values depends considerably on the past history of the patient.

Gas Exchange In Respiratory Failure

Patterns of Arterial Blood Gases

Various types of respiratory failure are associated with different degrees of hypoxemia and CO_2 retention. Figure 8.1 shows an O_2–CO_2 diagram with the line for a respiratory exchange ratio of 0.8. Pure hypoventilation leading to respiratory failure moves the arterial PO_2 and PCO_2 in the direction indicated by the *arrow* A. This pattern occurs in respiratory failure caused by neuromuscular disease, such as poliomyelitis, or by an overdose of a narcotic drug (Fig. 2.3). Severe ventilation–perfusion ratio inequality with alveolar ventilation inadequate to maintain a normal arterial PCO_2 results in movement along a line, such as B. The hypoxemia is more severe in relation to the hypercapnia than in the case of pure hypoventilation. Such a pattern is frequently seen in the respiratory failure of chronic obstructive pulmonary disease (COPD).

Severe interstitial disease sometimes results in movement along *line* C. Here there is increasingly severe hypoxemia but no CO_2 retention because of the raised ventilation. This pattern may be seen in advanced diffuse interstitial lung

Figure 8.1. **Patterns of arterial Po₂ and Pco₂ in different types of respiratory failure.**
Note that the Pco₂ can be high, as in pure hypoventilation *(A)*, or low, as in adult respiratory
distress syndrome *(D)*. The *broken lines* show the effects of oxygen breathing. (See text for
further details.)

disease or sarcoidosis. Sometimes there is a rise in arterial Pco₂, but this is
typically less marked than in obstructive diseases.

In respiratory failure caused by adult respiratory distress syndrome (ARDS),
the arterial Pco₂ is typically low, as shown by *line D*, but the hypoxemia may
be extreme. Such patients are usually treated with added inspired oxygen, which
raises the arterial Po₂ but often does not affect the Pco₂ (*D* to *E*) although in
some instances it may rise. Oxygen therapy to patients whose respiratory failure
is caused by COPD improves the arterial Po₂ but frequently causes a rise in Pco₂
because of depression of ventilation (*B* to *F*).

Hypoxemia of Respiratory Failure

Causes

Any of the four mechanisms of hypoxemia, hypoventilation, diffusion impairment, shunt, and ventilation–perfusion inequality, can contribute to the severe
hypoxemia of respiratory failure. However, the most important cause by far is
ventilation–perfusion inequality (including blood flow through unventilated
lung). This mechanism is largely responsible for the low arterial Po₂ in respiratory
failure complicating obstructive diseases, restrictive diseases, and ARDS.

Detection

Severe hypoxemia causes cyanosis, cardiovascular signs such as tachycardia, and
central nervous system effects such as mental confusion. However, a discussion
of the detection of hypoxemia from these signs is largely academic because
measurement of the Po₂ in the arterial blood is essential in determining the
degree of hypoxemia in patients with suspected respiratory failure.

Tissue Hypoxia

Hypoxemia is dangerous because it causes tissue hypoxia. However, the arterial Po_2 is only one factor in the delivery of oxygen to the tissues. Other factors include the oxygen capacity of the blood, the oxygen affinity of the hemoglobin, cardiac output, and the distribution of blood flow.

Tissues vary considerably in their vulnerability to hypoxia. Those at greatest risk include the central nervous system and the myocardium. Cessation of blood flow to the cerebral cortex results in loss of function within 4–6 seconds, loss of consciousness in 10–20 seconds, and irreversible changes in 3–5 minutes.

If the Po_2 falls below a critical level in tissue, aerobic oxidation ceases and anaerobic glycolysis takes over with the formation and release of increasing amounts of lactic acid. The Po_2 at which this occurs is not accurately known and probably varies between tissues. However, there is evidence that the critical intracellular Po_2 is of the order of 1 mm Hg in the region of the mitochondria.

Anaerobic glycolysis is a relatively inefficient method of obtaining energy from glucose. Nevertheless, it plays a critical role in maintaining tissue viability in respiratory failure. The large amounts of lactic acid that are formed are released into the blood, causing a metabolic acidosis. If tissue oxygenation subsequently improves, the lactic acid can be reconverted to glucose or used directly for energy. Most of this reconversion takes place in the liver.

Effects of Severe Hypoxemia

Mild hypoxemia produces few physiologic changes. It should be recalled that the arterial oxygen saturation is still approximately 90% when the Po_2 is only 60 mm Hg at a normal pH (Fig. 2.2). The only abnormalities are a slight impairment of mental performance and visual acuity and perhaps mild hyperventilation.

When the arterial Po_2 drops quickly below 40–50 mm Hg, deleterious effects are seen in several organ systems. The central nervous system is particularly vulnerable, and the patient often has headache, somnolence, or clouding of consciousness. Profound acute hypoxemia may cause convulsions, retinal hemorrhages, and permanent brain damage. The cardiovascular system shows tachycardia and mild hypertension, partly caused by the release of catecholamines; in severe hypoxemia there may be bradycardia and hypotension. Signs of heart failure may occur if there is associated coronary heart disease. Renal function is impaired, and sodium retention and proteinuria may be seen. Pulmonary hypertension is common because of the associated alveolar hypoxia.

Hypercapnia in Respiratory Failure

Causes

Both of the two mechanisms of CO_2 retention–hypoventilation and ventilation–perfusion inequality–can be important in respiratory failure. Hypoventilation is the cause in respiratory failure resulting from neuromuscular diseases such as the

Guillain-Barré syndrome, drug overdosage such as barbiturate poisoning, or a chest wall abnormality such as crushed chest (Fig. 2.4). Ventilation–perfusion inequality is the culprit in severe COPD and long-standing interstitial disease.

An important cause of CO_2 retention in respiratory failure is the injudicious use of oxygen therapy. Many patients with COPD gradually develop severe hypoxemia and some CO_2 retention over a period of months. It is not customary to refer to this situation as respiratory failure because these patients can continue in this state for long periods. However, such a patient usually has a high work of breathing (Figs. 3.3B and 4.12), and much of the ventilatory drive comes from hypoxic stimulation of the peripheral chemoreceptors. The arterial pH is virtually normal because of renal retention of bicarbonate (compensated respiratory acidosis), and the pH of the CSF is also normal because of an increase in bicarbonate there. Thus, despite an increased arterial Pco_2, the main ventilatory drive comes from the hypoxemia.

If this patient develops a relatively mild intercurrent respiratory infection and is treated with a high inspired oxygen concentration, a potentially dangerous situation can rapidly develop. The hypoxic ventilatory drive may be abolished while the work of breathing is increased because of retained secretions or bronchospasm. As a result, the ventilation may become grossly depressed and high levels of arterial Pco_2 may develop. In addition, profound hypoxemia may ensue if the oxygen is discontinued. This is because even if the ventilation does return to its previous level, the patient may take many minutes to unload the large accumulation of CO_2 in his or her tissues because of the large body stores of this gas.

A secondary cause of CO_2 retention in these patients may be the release of hypoxic vasoconstriction in poorly ventilated areas of lung as a result of the increased alveolar Po_2. The consequences of this are increased blood flow to low $\dot{V}A/\dot{Q}$ areas and a worsening of $\dot{V}A/\dot{Q}$ inequality that exaggerates the CO_2 retention. This factor is probably less important than the depression of ventilation, but the rapid rise in arterial Pco_2 that is seen when some of these patients are given oxygen suggests that this mechanism may play a part.

Such patients present a therapeutic dilemma. On the one hand, oxygen administration is likely to cause severe CO_2 retention and respiratory acidosis. On the other hand, it is clearly essential to give some oxygen to relieve the life-threatening hypoxemia. The answer to this problem is to give a relatively low concentration (24–28% O_2) and to monitor the arterial blood gases frequently to determine whether depression of ventilation is occurring. Intubation and mechanical ventilation may become necessary. The use of added oxygen is discussed further in Chapter 9.

Effects

Raised levels of Pco_2 in the blood greatly increase cerebral blood flow, causing headache, raised CSF pressure, and, sometimes, papilledema. In practice, the cerebral effects of hypercapnia overlap with the effects of hypoxemia. The resulting abnormalities include restlessness, tremor, slurred speech, asterixis (flapping tremor), and fluctuations of mood. High levels of P_{CO_2} are narcotic and cause clouding of consciousness.

Acidosis in Respiratory Failure

The CO_2 retention causes a respiratory acidosis that may be severe, especially after the injudicious administration of oxygen. However, patients who gradually develop respiratory failure may retain considerable amounts of bicarbonate, keeping the fall of pH in check (Fig. 2.11).

Metabolic acidosis frequently coexists with respiratory acidosis and complicates the acid–base abnormality. This is caused by the liberation of lactic acid from hypoxic tissues, and the dual factors of hypoxemia and an inadequate peripheral circulation are additive. In patients who are mechanically ventilated, the raised intrathoracic pressure may interfere with venous return and cardiac output and thus further reduce peripheral blood flow (Fig. 10.6).

Role of Diaphragm Fatigue

Fatigue of the diaphragm can contribute to the hypoventilation of respiratory failure. The diaphragm consists of striated skeletal muscle controlled by voluntary and automatic neural pathways via the phrenic nerves. Although the diaphragm is predominantly made up of slow twitch oxidative fibers and fast twitch oxidative glycolytic fibers, which are relatively resistant to fatigue, this can occur if the work of breathing is greatly increased over prolonged periods of time. Fatigue can be defined as a loss of contractile force after work, and can be measured from the transdiaphragmatic pressure resulting from a maximum contraction, or indirectly from the muscle relaxation time or the electromyogram. There is evidence that some patients with severe COPD continually breathe close to the work level at which fatigue occurs, and that an exacerbation of infection can tip them over into a fatigue state. This will then result in hypoventilation, CO_2 retention, and severe hypoxemia. Because hypercapnia impairs diaphragm contractility and severe hypoxemia accelerates the onset of fatigue, a vicious circle develops.

The dangers of diaphragm fatigue can be limited by reducing the work of breathing by treating bronchospasm and controlling infection, and by giving oxygen judiciously to relieve the hypoxemia. The force of contraction can be improved by a training program, for example, by breathing through inspiratory resistances. In addition, the administration of methylxanthines improves diaphragm contractility and, because these drugs also relieve reversible bronchoconstriction, they are frequently useful. However, the role of fatigue of the diaphragm in respiratory failure is still not fully understood.

Types of Respiratory Failure

A large number of conditions can lead to respiratory failure, and various classifications are possible. However, from the point of view of the physiological principles of management, five groups can be distinguished:

1. Acute overwhelming lung disease
2. Neuromuscular disorders
3. Acute on chronic lung disease
4. Adult respiratory distress syndrome
5. Infant respiratory distress syndrome

Acute Overwhelming Lung Disease

Many acute diseases, if severe enough, can lead to respiratory failure. These include infections such as fulminating viral or bacterial pneumonias, vascular diseases such as pulmonary embolism, and exposure to inhaled toxic substances such as chlorine gas or oxides of nitrogen. Respiratory failure supervenes as the primary disease progresses, and profound hypoxemia with or without hypercapnia develops. Oxygen administration is required for the hypoxemia, and mechanical ventilation may be necessary to tide the patient over the worst stage. A few patients have been treated by extracorporeal membrane oxygenators that largely take over the gas exchange function of the lung. Treatment of the underlying disease, for example, antibiotics for bacterial pneumonias, clearly is necessary. This group of conditions merges into ARDS (see later text).

Neuromuscular Disorders

Respiratory failure may occur when the respiratory center is depressed by drugs such as heroin and barbiturates. Other conditions include central nervous system and neuromuscular diseases such as encephalitis, poliomyelitis, Guillain-Barré syndrome, myasthenia gravis, anticholinesterase poisoning, amyotrophic lateral sclerosis, and progressive muscular dystrophy (Fig. 2.4). Trauma to the chest wall also can be responsible.

In these conditions, the essential feature is hypoventilation leading to CO_2 retention with moderate hypoxemia (Figs. 2.3 and 8.1). Respiratory acidosis occurs, but the magnitude of the fall in pH depends on the rapidity of the increase in Pco_2 and the extent of the renal compensation.

Mechanical ventilation is often necessary in these conditions and occasionally, as in bulbar poliomyelitis, it may be required for months or even years. However, the lung itself is often normal and, if so, no additional oxygen is necessary to reverse the hypoxemia. Again, treatment of the underlying disease is always indicated, if available.

Acute on Chronic Lung Disease

This is an important and common group that includes patients with chronic bronchitis and emphysema, asthma, and cystic fibrosis. Many patients with COPD follow a gradual downhill course with increasingly severe hypoxemia and CO_2 retention over months or years. Such patients are usually capable of limited physical activity even though both the arterial Po_2 and Pco_2 may be in the region of 50 mm Hg. As a result, this situation is not conventionally referred to as respiratory failure.

However, if such a patient develops even a mild exacerbation of his chest infection, his or her condition often deteriorates rapidly, with profound hypoxemia, CO_2 retention, and respiratory acidosis. The reserves of pulmonary function are minimal, and any increase in the work of breathing or worsening of ventilation–perfusion relationships as a result of retained secretions or bronchospasm pushes the patient over the brink into frank respiratory failure.

The management of these patients requires a delicate touch. Naturally, the underlying infection should be treated with antibiotics. In addition, bronchodilators may be indicated for bronchospasm, and diuretics and digitalis may be required if there is evidence of heart failure. Supplemental oxygen is necessary to relieve the severe hypoxemia. However, these patients frequently lose their ventilatory drive and develop severe CO_2 retention and acidosis if too much oxygen is administered. For this reason, it is usual to begin with 24–28% oxygen and monitor the arterial blood gases frequently (see Chapter 9).

Mechanical ventilation may be necessary, but the decision to employ this is often a difficult one. On the one hand, it may be impossible to prevent the rise of arterial P_{CO_2} without artificial ventilation. On the other hand, these patients often have such diseased lungs that, once they are on the ventilator, it may be difficult or impossible to wean them from it. Each case must be considered on its own merits, but mechanical ventilation should generally be used only if there is a substantial reversible component to the patient's condition.

Adult Respiratory Distress Syndrome

This condition is sometimes referred to as "acute respiratory failure." It is an end result of a variety of insults, including trauma to the lung or to the rest of the body, aspiration, sepsis (especially that caused by gram-negative organisms), and shock from any cause (40). There is evidence that many other organs are also affected, and the condition should probably be regarded as multi-organ failure.

Pathology

The early changes consist of interstitial and alveolar edema. Hemorrhage, cellular debris, and proteinaceous fluid are present in the alveoli, hyaline membranes may be seen, and there is patchy atelectasis (Fig. 8.2). Later, hyperplasia and organization occur. The damaged alveolar epithelium becomes lined with type 2 alveolar cells, and there is cellular infiltration of the alveolar walls. Eventually, interstitial fibrosis may develop, although complete healing can occur.

Pathogenesis

This is still unclear and many factors may play a role (41). The capillary endothelial and type I alveolar epithelial cells are damaged early, causing increased capillary permeability and flooding of the alveoli with proteinaceous fluid. Neutrophils accumulate partly as a result of complement or kinin activation. The activated neutrophils release mediators, including bradykinin, histamine, and platelet activating factor (PAF). In addition, toxic oxygen radicals are generated, together with cyclooxygenase products such as prostaglandins and thromboxane,

Figure 8.2.   Histologic changes in adult respiratory distress syndrome as found by an open lung biopsy. There are patchy atelectasis, edema, hyaline membranes, and cellular debris in the alveoli. (From Lamy M, Fallat RJ, Koeniger E, et al. Pathologic features and mechanisms of hypoxemia in adult respiratory distress syndrome. Am Rev Resp Dis 1976;114:267–284.)

and also lipoxygenase products such as leukotrienes. Platelets activated by PAF release proteases and kallikrein.

Clinical Features

ARDS is often associated with some severe underlying medical or surgical illness unconnected with the lung, and the onset of respiratory failure is often delayed. A typical history is that the patient is exposed to severe trauma, for example, an automobile accident with multiple fractures. There is some hemorrhagic shock with hypotension that is treated by fluid replacement. The patient appears to be doing well when, perhaps 2 days after the trauma, some increase in respiratory rate is noted, the arterial Po_2 and Pco_2 fall, and clouding is seen in the chest radiograph, which progresses to dense uneven opacification. Severe hypoxemia develops. The mortality rate is approximately 50%.

Pulmonary Function

The lung becomes very stiff, and unusually high pressures are required to ventilate it mechanically. Associated with this reduced compliance is a marked fall in FRC. The cause of the increased recoil is presumably the alveolar edema and exudate, which exaggerate the surface tension forces. As was pointed out earlier

Figure 8.3. **Distribution of ventilation–perfusion ratios in a patient who developed adult respiratory distress syndrome after an automobile accident.** Note the 8% shunt and the blood flow to units with low ventilation–perfusion ratios. In addition, there is some ventilation to high V̇A/Q̇ units, probably as a result of the high airway pressure developed by the ventilator (compare Fig. 10.4).

(Fig. 6.3), edematous alveoli have a reduced volume. It is also possible that interstitial edema contributes to the abnormal stiffness of the lungs.

As would be expected from the histologic appearance of the lung (Fig. 8.2), there is marked ventilation–perfusion inequality, with a substantial fraction of the total blood flow going to unventilated alveoli. This fraction may reach 50% or more. Figure 8.3 shows some results obtained by the multiple inert gas method in a 44-year-old patient who developed respiratory failure after an automobile accident and who was mechanically ventilated. Note the presence of blood flow to lung units with abnormally low ventilation–perfusion ratios and also the shunt of 8% (compare the normal distribution in Fig. 2.9). Figure 8.3 also shows a large amount of ventilation going to units with high ventilation–perfusion ratios. One reason for this is the abnormally high airway pressures developed by the ventilator, which reduces the blood flow in some alveoli (compare Fig. 10.4).

The ventilation–perfusion inequality and shunt cause profound hypoxemia. These patients usually must be given oxygen-enriched mixtures because air breathing, even with a ventilator, results in an arterial Po_2 which is dangerously low. Oxygen concentrations of 40–100% are sometimes necessary during mechanical ventilation to maintain an arterial Po_2 above 60 mm Hg. However, the possibility of oxygen toxicity should be kept in mind (Chapter 9). The addition of positive end-expiratory pressure (PEEP) often results in a substantial improvement in oxygenation in these patients (compare Fig. 10.4).

By contrast, the arterial Pco_2 is typically low, even when severe hypoxemia develops; values in the 20s are common. The reason for the increased ventilation is not known, although possibly the interstitial edema stimulates intrapulmonary J or stretch receptors. Another possible factor is stimulation of the peripheral chemoreceptors by the hypoxemia, although relieving this usually does not affect the level of ventilation.

Infant Respiratory Distress Syndrome

This condition, which is also called hyaline membrane disease of the newborn, has several features in common with ARDS (43). Pathologically, the lung shows hemorrhagic edema, patchy atelectasis, and hyaline membranes caused by proteinaceous fluid and cellular debris within the alveoli. Physiologically, there is profound hypoxemia, with both ventilation–perfusion inequality and blood flow through unventilated lung. In addition, a right-to-left shunt via the patent foramen ovale may exaggerate the hypoxemia. Mechanical ventilation with enriched oxygen mixtures is often necessary, and the addition of PEEP or continuous positive airway pressure (see Chapter 10) is frequently beneficial.

The chief cause of this condition is an absence of pulmonary surfactant, although other factors are probably also involved. The surfactant is normally produced by the type 2 alveolar cells (Fig. 5.2), and the ability of the lung to synthesize adequate amounts of the material develops relatively late in fetal life. Thus, a prematurely born infant is particularly at risk. The ability of the infant to secrete surfactant can be estimated by measuring the lecithin/sphingomyelin ratio of amniotic fluid, and that maturation of the surfactant-synthesizing system can be hastened by the administration of corticosteroids. Treatment of the condition by administering exogenous surfactant via the trachea is now valuable.

Management of Respiratory Failure

Although many factors enter into the management of an individual patient, it is useful to discuss the physiologic principles that underlie treatment. Naturally, attention must be directed to the primary cause of the disease. For example, antibiotic therapy may be required for an infection, or a specific treatment may be available for a neuromuscular disorder. However, some aspects of management are common to many patients with respiratory failure.

Airway Obstruction

Respiratory failure is often precipitated by an increase in airway resistance. Many patients have COPD of many years' duration with hypoxemia and even some mild hypercapnia. Even so, they are able to maintain some physical activity. However, if they develop bronchospasm through exposure to smog or cold air or if they have a "chesty cold" with an increase in secretions, they may rapidly develop respiratory failure. The additional work of breathing becomes the straw that breaks the camel's back, and they develop profound hypoxemia, CO_2 retention, and respiratory acidosis.

Treatment should be directed at reducing the airway obstruction. Retained secretions are best removed by coughing when this is effective. Encouragement to cough and assistance by a respiratory therapist, nurse, or physician is often helpful, and changing the patient's position from side to side to assist drainage of secretions may be beneficial. Adequate hydration is important to prevent the secretions from becoming too viscid. It is especially important to humidify all gases given by a ventilator to prevent thickening and crusting of secretions. Drugs such as potassium iodide by mouth or acetylcysteine by aerosol to liquefy sputum are of doubtful value. Chest physiotherapy may help to clear airway secretions. However, aspiration of secretions by bronchoscopy may become necessary. Occasionally, respiratory stimulants are given to a drowsy patient but, more importantly, respiratory depressants must be avoided because they suppress coughing.

Any reversible airway obstruction should be treated by bronchodilators, such as albuterol or metaproterenol aerosol, intravenous aminophylline, or perhaps intravenous corticosteroids. Drugs such as isoproterenol that also stimulate β_1-adrenergic receptors in the heart should be avoided.

Respiratory Infection

An exacerbation of existing bronchitis in a patient with COPD, or a fresh respiratory infection in a patient with advanced interstitial lung disease, frequently provokes respiratory failure. There are at least two physiologic mechanisms for this. First, the increased secretions and, perhaps, bronchospasm increase the work of breathing as discussed earlier. Second, there is a worsening of ventilation–perfusion relationships, so that even if the ventilation to the alveoli remains unchanged, there will be increasing hypoxemia and hypercapnia. Treatment of the infection by antibiotics is indicated.

Even a mild exacerbation of bronchitis in a patient with COPD may precipitate respiratory failure. Moreover, the usual systemic responses to infection, such as pyrexia and leukocytosis, are often absent. However, treatment should not be delayed.

Cardiac Insufficiency

Many patients with incipient respiratory failure have a compromised cardiovascular system. The pulmonary artery pressure is raised frequently as a result of several factors, including destruction of the pulmonary capillary bed by disease, hypoxic vasoconstriction, and increased blood viscosity caused by polycythemia. In addition, the myocardium is chronically hypoxic. Fluid retention often occurs as a result of retention of bicarbonate and sodium ions by the hypoxic kidney. Finally, some patients have coexisting coronary artery disease.

Patients with COPD frequently develop peripheral edema, hepatomegaly, and engorged neck veins. These and other patients may also show signs of left heart failure, with basal rales (crackles) on auscultation and engorged lung fields on the radiograph. The mild pulmonary edema further interferes with pulmonary gas exchange by causing uneven ventilation. Treatment with diuretics and digitalis is then indicated.

Hypoxemia

Hypoxemia can be relieved to some extent by treating the airway obstruction and the chest infection. However, the administration of long-term oxygen is frequently required, and this important topic is discussed in detail in Chapter 9.

Hypercapnia

Hypercapnia often responds to general measures directed at the airway obstruction and the infection. However, mechanical ventilation is frequently required. This is discussed in detail in Chapter 10.

9   Oxygen Therapy

Oxygen administration has a critical role in the treatment of hypoxemia and, especially, in the management of respiratory failure. However, patients vary considerably in their response to oxygen, and there are several potential hazards associated with its use. A clear understanding of the physiologic principles involved is necessary to prevent abuses of this powerful agent.

Improved Oxygenation After Oxygen Administration

Power of Added Oxygen

The great extent to which the arterial Po_2 can be increased by the inhalation of 100% oxygen is sometimes not appreciated. Suppose a young man has taken an overdose of a narcotic drug that results in severe hypoventilation with an arterial Po_2 of 50 and a Pco_2 of 80 mm Hg (Fig. 2.3). If this patient is mechanically ventilated and given 100% oxygen, the arterial Po_2 may increase to over 600 mm Hg; that is a 10-fold increase (Fig. 9.1). Few drugs can change the gas exchange of the blood so greatly and so effortlessly!

Response of Various Types of Hypoxemia

The mechanism of hypoxemia has an important bearing on its response to inhaled oxygen.

Hypoventilation

The rise in alveolar Po_2 can be predicted from the alveolar gas equation *if* the ventilation and metabolic rate, and therefore the alveolar Pco_2, remain unaltered:

Figure 9.1.   Response of the arterial Po₂ to 100% inspired oxygen for the different mechanisms of hypoxemia. The Po₂ breathing air is assumed to be 50 mm Hg. Note the dramatic increase in all instances except shunt where, nevertheless, there is a useful gain.

$$P_{A_{O_2}} = P_{I_{O_2}} - \frac{P_{A_{CO_2}}}{R} + F \qquad\qquad (Eq.\ 9.1)$$

where F is a small correction factor.

Assuming no change in the alveolar P_{CO_2} and the respiratory exchange ratio and neglecting the correction factor, this equation shows that the alveolar P_{O_2} rises parallel with the inspired value. Thus changing from air to only 30% oxygen can increase the alveolar P_{O_2} by approximately 60 mm Hg. In practice, the arterial P_{O_2} is always lower than the alveolar value because of a small amount of venous admixture. However, the hypoxemia of hypoventilation, which is rarely severe (Fig. 2.3), is easily reversed by a modest oxygen enrichment of the inspired gas.

Diffusion Impairment

Again, hypoxemia caused by this mechanism is readily overcome by oxygen administration. The reason for this becomes clear if we look at the dynamics of oxygen uptake along the pulmonary capillary (Fig. 2.5). The rate of movement of oxygen across the blood–gas barrier is proportional to the P_{O_2} difference between alveolar gas and capillary blood. (See West JB. Respiratory physiology–the essentials, ed. 5. Baltimore: Williams & Wilkins, 1995: p. 24.) This difference is normally approximately 60 mm Hg at the beginning of the capillary. If we increase the concentration of inspired oxygen to only 30%, we raise the alveolar P_{O_2} by 60 mm Hg, thus doubling the rate of transfer of oxygen at the start of the capillary. This in turn improves oxygenation of the end-capillary blood. Therefore, a modest rise in inspired oxygen concentration can usually correct the hypoxemia.

Ventilation–perfusion Inequality

Again, oxygen administration usually is very effective at improving the arterial P_{O_2}. However, the rise in P_{O_2} depends on the pattern of ventilation–perfusion inequality and the inspired oxygen concentration. Administration of 100% O_2 increases the arterial P_{O_2} to very high values because every lung unit that is ventilated eventually washes out its nitrogen. When this occurs, the alveolar P_{O_2} is given by $P_{O_2} = P_B - P_{H_2O} - P_{CO_2}$. Because the P_{CO_2} is normally less than 50 mm Hg, this equation predicts an alveolar P_{O_2} of over 600 mm Hg, even in lung units with very low ventilation–perfusion ratios.

However, two cautions should be added. First, some regions of the lung may be so poorly ventilated that it may take many minutes for the nitrogen to be washed out. Furthermore, these regions may continue to receive nitrogen as this gas is gradually washed out of peripheral tissues by the venous blood. As a consequence, the arterial P_{O_2} may take so long to reach its final level that in practice this is never achieved. Second, giving oxygen may result in the development of unventilated areas (Fig. 9.5). If this occurs, the rise in arterial P_{O_2} stops short (Fig. 9.3).

When intermediate concentrations of oxygen are given, the rise in arterial P_{O_2} is determined by the pattern of ventilation–perfusion inequality and in particular by those units that have low ventilation–perfusion ratios and appreciable blood flow. Figure 9.2 shows the response of the arterial P_{O_2} in lung models

Figure 9.2.   Response of the arterial P_{O_2} to various inspired oxygen values in theoretical distributions of ventilation–perfusion ratios. SD refers to the standard deviation of the log normal distribution. Note that when the distribution is broad (SD = 2), the arterial P_{O_2} remains low even when 60% oxygen is inhaled. (From West JB, Wagner PD. Pulmonary gas exchange. In: West JB. ed. Bioengineering aspects of the lung. New York: Marcel Dekker, 1977.)

with various distributions of ventilation–perfusion ratios after inspiration of various oxygen concentrations (44). Note that at an inspired concentration of 60%, the arterial Po_2 of the distribution with a standard deviation of 2.0 rose from 40 to only 90 mm Hg. This modest rise can be attributed to the effects of lung units with ventilation–perfusion ratios less than 0.01. For example, an alveolus with a ventilation–perfusion ratio of 0.006 that is given 60% O_2 to inspire has an end-capillary Po_2 of only 60 mm Hg in the example shown. However, note that when the inspired oxygen concentration was increased to 90%, the arterial Po_2 of this distribution rose to nearly 500 mm Hg.

Figure 9.2 assumes that the pattern of ventilation–perfusion inequality re-mains constant as the inspired oxygen is raised. However, the relief of alveolar hypoxia in poorly ventilated regions of lung may increase the blood flow there because of the abolition of hypoxic vasoconstriction. In this case, the increase in arterial Po_2 will be less. Note also that if units with low ventilation–perfusion ratios collapse during high oxygen breathing (Figs. 9.5 and 9.6), the arterial Po_2 rises less.

Shunt

This is the only mechanism of hypoxemia in which the arterial Po_2 remains far below the level for the normal lung during 100% O_2 breathing. The reason is that the blood that bypasses the ventilated alveoli (shunt) does not "see" the added oxygen and, being low in oxygen concentration, depresses the arterial Po_2. This depression is particularly marked because of the shallow slope of the oxygen dissociation curve at a high Po_2 (Fig. 2.7).

However, it should be emphasized that useful gains in arterial Po_2 often follow the administration of 100% O_2 to patients with shunts. This is because of the additional dissolved oxygen which can be appreciable at a high alveolar Po_2. For example, increasing the alveolar Po_2 from 100 to 600 mm Hg raises the dissolved oxygen in the end capillary blood from 0.3 to 1.8 ml of O_2/100 ml of blood. This increase of 1.5 can be compared with the normal arterial–venous difference in oxygen concentration of approximately 5 ml/100 ml.

Figure 9.3 shows typical increases in arterial Po_2 for various percentage shunts at different inspired oxygen concentrations. The graph is drawn for an oxygen uptake of 300 ml/min and cardiac output of 6 liters/min; variations in these and other values alter the positions of the lines. However, in this example, a patient with a 30% shunt who has an arterial Po_2 of 55 mm Hg during air breathing increases this to 110 mm Hg if he or she breathes 100% oxygen. This increase corresponds to a rise in oxygen saturation and concentration of the arterial blood of 10% and 2.2 ml/100 ml, respectively. In a patient with a hypoxic myocardium, for example, these values mean an important gain in oxygen delivery.

Other Factors in Oxygen Delivery

Although the arterial Po_2 is a convenient measurement of the degree of oxygen-ation of the blood, other factors are important in oxygen delivery to the tissues. These factors include the hemoglobin concentration, the position of the oxygen

Figure 9.3. Response of the arterial Po₂ to increased inspired oxygen concentrations in a lung with various amounts of shunt. Note that the Po₂ remains a long way below the normal level for 100% oxygen. Nevertheless, useful gains in oxygenation occur even with severe degrees of shunting. (This diagram shows typical values only; changes in cardiac output, oxygen uptake, etc., affect the position of the lines.)

dissociation curve, the cardiac output, and the distribution of the blood flow throughout the peripheral tissues.

Both a fall in hemoglobin concentration and cardiac output reduce the total amount of oxygen per unit time (*"oxygen flux"*) going to the tissues. The flux may be expressed as the product of the cardiac output and the arterial oxygen concentration: $\dot{Q} \times Ca_{O_2}$.

Diffusion of oxygen from the peripheral capillaries to the mitochondria in the tissue cells depends on capillary Po₂. A useful index is the Po₂ of mixed venous blood, which is close to the average tissue Po₂. A rearrangement of the Fick equation is as follows:

$$C\bar{v}_{O_2} = Ca_{O_2} - \frac{\dot{V}_{O_2}}{\dot{Q}}$$ (Eq. 9.2)

This equation shows that the oxygen concentration (and therefore the Po₂) of mixed venous blood will fall if either the arterial oxygen concentration or the cardiac output is reduced (oxygen consumption assumed constant).

The relationship between oxygen concentration and Po₂ in the mixed venous blood depends on the position of the oxygen dissociation curve (Fig. 2.2). If the curve is shifted to the right by an increase in temperature, as in fever, or an increase in 2,3-DPG concentration, as frequently occurs in chronic hypoxemia, the Po₂ for a given content is high, thus favoring diffusion of oxygen to the mitochondria. By contrast if the Pco₂ is low and the pH is high, as in respiratory alkalosis, or if the 2,3-DPG concentration is low because of transfusion of large amounts of stored blood, the resulting left-shifted curve interferes with oxygen unloading to the tissues.

Finally, the distribution of cardiac output clearly plays an important role in tissue oxygenation. For example, a patient who has coronary artery disease is liable to have hypoxic regions in the myocardium, irrespective of the other factors involved in oxygen delivery.

Methods of Oxygen Administration

Nasal Cannulas

Nasal cannulas consist of two prongs that are inserted just inside the anterior nares and supported on a light frame. Oxygen is supplied at rates of 1–4 liters/min, resulting in inspired oxygen concentrations of approximately 25–30%. The higher the patient's inspiratory flow rate, the lower the resulting concentration. The gas should be humidified as close to body temperature as possible to prevent crusting of secretions on the nasal mucosa.

The chief advantage of cannulas is that the patient does not have the discomfort of a mask and he or she can talk and eat and has access to the face. The cannulas can be worn continuously for long periods, an important point because oxygen administration should usually be continuous rather than intermittent (see later text). The disadvantages of cannulas are the low maximum inspired concentrations of oxygen that are available and the unpredictability of the concentration, especially if the patient breathes mostly through his or her mouth.

Masks

Masks come in several designs. Simple plastic masks that fit over the nose and mouth allow inspired oxygen concentrations of up to 60% when supplied with flow rates of 6 liters/min. However, because some accumulation of CO_2 occurs within the mask (up to 2%), this device should be used with caution in patients who are liable to develop CO_2 retention. In addition, some patients report feeling smothered when this type of mask is used.

A useful mask for delivering controlled oxygen concentrations is based on the Venturi principle. As the oxygen enters the mask through a narrow jet, it entrains a constant flow of air, which enters via surrounding holes. With an oxygen flow of 4 liters/min, a total flow(oxygen + air) of approximately 40 liters/min is delivered to the patient. At such high flow rates, there is negligible rebreathing of expired gas and, therefore, no CO_2 accumulation. Masks that give inspired oxygen concentrations of 24, 28, or 35% with a high degree of reliability are available and are particularly useful for treating patients who are liable to develop CO_2 retention. Some patients complain of the noise and the breeze, while others enjoy the latter.

Transtracheal Oxygen

This can be delivered via a microcatheter inserted through the anterior tracheal wall with the tip lying just above the carina. It is an efficient way of delivering oxygen, particularly for patients on long-term oxygen therapy, although care must be taken to prevent infection.

Tents

These are now used only for children who do not tolerate masks well: Oxygen concentrations of up to 50% can be obtained.

Ventilators

When a patient is mechanically ventilated through an endotracheal or tracheostomy tube, complete control over the composition of the inspired gas is available. Danger of producing oxygen toxicity exists if concentrations of over 50% are given for more than 2 days (see later text). In general, the lowest inspired oxygen that provides an acceptable arterial P_{O_2} should be used. This level is difficult to define, but in patients with ARDS who are being mechanically ventilated with high oxygen concentrations, a figure of 60 mm Hg is often used.

Hyperbaric Oxygen

If 100% O_2 is administered at a pressure of 3 atmospheres, the inspired P_{O_2} is over 2000 mm Hg. Under these conditions, a substantial increase in the arterial oxygen concentration can occur, chiefly as a result of additional dissolved oxygen. For example, if the arterial P_{O_2} is 2000 mm Hg, the oxygen in solution is approximately 6 ml/100 ml of blood. Theoretically, this is enough to provide the entire arterial–venous difference of 5 ml/100 ml, so that the hemoglobin of the mixed venous blood could remain fully saturated.

Hyperbaric oxygen therapy has limited uses and is rarely indicated in the management of respiratory failure. However, it has been used in the treatment of severe carbon monoxide poisoning in which most of the hemoglobin is unavailable to carry oxygen and therefore, the dissolved oxygen is critically important. In addition, the high P_{O_2} accelerates the dissociation of carbon monoxide from hemoglobin. A severe anemic crisis is sometimes treated in the same way. Hyperbaric oxygen is also used in the treatment of gas gangrene infections and as an adjunct to radiotherapy where the higher tissue P_{O_2} increases the radiosensitivity of relatively avascular tumors. The high pressure chamber is also valuable for managing decompression sickness.

The use of hyperbaric oxygen requires a special facility with trained personnel. In practice, the chamber is filled with air and oxygen is given by a special mask to ensure that the patient receives pure oxygen. This procedure also reduces fire hazard.

Domiciliary and Portable Oxygen

Some patients are so disabled by severe chronic pulmonary disease that they are virtually confined to bed or a chair unless they breathe supplementary oxygen. These patients often benefit considerably from having a supply of oxygen in their home. This can take various forms. A central large tank with a long plastic tube and mask may enable the patient to climb stairs or go to the bathroom.

In addition, portable oxygen sets are available, and these can be used for shopping or other activities. Some sets use liquid oxygen as a store; these are best for patient mobility. In others, oxygen is extracted from the air with a molecular sieve.

The patients who benefit most from portable oxygen are those whose exercise tolerance is limited by dyspnea. Increasing the inspired oxygen concentration can greatly increase the level of exercise for a given ventilation and so enable these patients to become much more active.

It has been shown that a low flow of oxygen given continuously over several months can reduce the amount of pulmonary hypertension and improve the prognosis of some patients with advanced COPD. Although such therapy is expensive, improvements in the technology of providing oxygen have made it feasible.

Hazards of Oxygen Therapy

Carbon Dioxide Retention

The reasons for the development of dangerous CO_2 retention after oxygen administration to patients with severe COPD were briefly discussed on page 134. A critical factor in the ventilatory drive of these patients who have a high work of breathing is often the hypoxic stimulation of their peripheral chemoreceptors. If this is removed by relieving their hypoxemia, the level of ventilation may fall precipitously and severe CO_2 retention may ensue.

Intermittent oxygen therapy is especially dangerous. The physiologist Haldane compared this with bringing a drowning man to the surface–occasionally!

The explanation is that if oxygen administration is seen to cause CO_2 retention and is therefore stopped, the subsequent hypoxemia may be more severe than it was before oxygen therapy. The reason is the increased alveolar P_{CO_2} as can be seen from the alveolar gas equation:

$$P_{A_{O_2}} = P_{I_{O_2}} - \frac{P_{A_{CO_2}}}{R} + F \qquad \text{(Eq. 9.3)}$$

Moreover, the high P_{CO_2} is likely to remain for many minutes because the body stores of this gas are so great that the excess is washed out only gradually. Thus, the hypoxemia may be severe and prolonged.

These patients should be given continuous oxygen at a low concentration, and the blood gases must be monitored. Initially, an oxygen concentration of 24% is often given by means of a Venturi mask, and the arterial P_{O_2} and P_{CO_2} are measured after 15–20 minutes. If the P_{CO_2} does not rise more than a few mm Hg and the patient remains alert, the oxygen concentration can be increased to 28%. This is generally adequate to relieve severe hypoxemia, although concentrations as high as 35% are sometimes used. The shape of the oxygen dissociation curve (Fig. 2.2) should be at the back of the physician's mind to remind him or her that a rise in P_{O_2} from 30 to 50 mm Hg (at a normal pH) represents more than a 25% increase in hemoglobin saturation!

Oxygen Toxicity

High concentrations of oxygen over long periods damage the lung. Fig. 9.4 shows an electron micrograph from a monkey exposed to 100% oxygen for 2 days (compare Fig. 5.1) (45). Note the swollen capillary endothelium which is where some of the earliest changes are seen. Alterations also occur in the endothelial intercellular junctions, and there is an increased capillary permeability that leads to interstitial and alveolar edema. In addition, the alveolar epithelium may become completely denuded and replaced by rows of type 2 epithelial cells. Later, organization occurs, with interstitial fibrosis.

In humans, the pulmonary effects of high oxygen concentration are more difficult to document, but normal subjects report substernal discomfort after breathing 100% oxygen for 24 hours. Patients who have been mechanically ventilated with 100% oxygen for 36 hours have shown a progressive fall in arterial Po_2 compared with a control group who were ventilated with air. A reasonable attitude is to assume that concentrations of 50% or higher for more than 2 days may produce toxic changes.

In practice, such high levels over such a long period can only be achieved in patients who are intubated and mechanically ventilated. It is important to avoid oxygen toxicity because the only way to relieve the resultant hypoxemia is by raising the inspired oxygen, thus creating a vicious circle.

Atelectasis

Following Airway Occlusion

If a patient is breathing air and an airway becomes totally obstructed, for example, by retained secretions, absorption atelectasis of the lung behind the airway may occur. The reason is that the sum of the partial pressures in venous blood is considerably less than atmospheric pressure, with the result that the trapped gas is gradually absorbed. (See West JB. Respiratory physiology–the essentials, ed. 5. Baltimore: Williams & Wilkins, 1995: p. 141.) However, the process is relatively slow, requiring many hours or even days.

However, if the patient is breathing a high concentration of oxygen, the rate of absorption atelectasis is greatly accelerated. This is because there is then relatively little nitrogen in the alveoli and this gas normally slows the absorption process because of its low solubility. Replacing the nitrogen with any other gas that is rapidly absorbed also predisposes to collapse. An example is nitrous oxide during anesthesia. In the normal lung, collateral ventilation may delay or prevent atelectasis by providing an alternate path for gas to enter the obstructed region (Fig. 1.12C).

Absorption atelectasis is common in patients with respiratory failure because they often have excessive secretions or cellular debris in their airways and they are frequently treated with high oxygen concentrations. In addition, the channels through which collateral ventilation normally occurs may be obstructed by disease. Collapse is common in the dependent regions of the lung because secretions tend to collect there, and those airways and alveoli are relatively

Figure 9.4. Early changes in oxygen toxicity. This electron micrograph from a monkey exposed to 100% oxygen for 2 days shows swelling of the capillary endothelial cells. Later changes include loss of alveolar epithelium and subsequent interstitial fibrosis. *A*, alveolus; *EN*, endothelium, *EP*, epithelium; *IN*, interstitium; *RBC*, red blood cell. (From Kapanci U, Weibel ER, Kaplan HP, et al. Pathogenesis and reversibility of the pulmonary lesions of oxygen toxicity in monkeys. Lab Invest 1969;20:101–118.)

poorly expanded anyway (Fig. 3.5). To the extent that atelectatic lung is perfused, hypoxemia develops, although hypoxic vasoconstriction may limit this to some extent.

Instability of Units with Low Ventilation–Perfusion Ratios

It has been shown that lung units with low ventilation–perfusion ratios may become unstable and collapse when high oxygen mixtures are inhaled. An example is given in Figure 9.5, which shows the distribution of ventilation–perfusion ratios in a patient during air breathing and after 30 minutes of 100% oxygen. This patient had respiratory failure after an automobile accident (Fig. 8.3). Note that during air breathing there were appreciable amounts of blood flow to lung units with low ventilation–perfusion ratios in addition to an 8% shunt. After oxygen administration, the blood flow to the low ventilation–perfusion ratio units was not evident, but the shunt had increased to 16%. The most likely explanation of this change is that the poorly ventilated regions became unventilated.

Figure 9.6 shows the mechanism involved. The figure shows four hypothetical lung units, all with low inspired ventilation–perfusion ratios ($\dot{V}$AI/$\dot{Q}$) during 80% oxygen breathing. In A, the inspired (alveolar) ventilation is 49.4 units but the expired ventilation is only 2.5 units (the actual values depend on the

Figure 9.5. Conversion of low ventilation–perfusion ratio units to shunt during oxygen breathing. This patient had respiratory failure after an automobile accident (same patient as shown in Figure 8.3). During air breathing there was appreciable blood flow to units with low ventilation–perfusion ratios. After 30 minutes of 100% oxygen, blood flow to these units was not evident, but the shunt doubled.

Inspired $O_2 = 80\%$

$\dot{V}_{AI}/\dot{Q}$ 0.0494   0.0440   0.0373   0.0373

49.4 → 2.5   44.0   37.3 ~ 2.0   37.3

Stable   Critical   Unstable

A   B   C   D

Figure 9.6.   Mechanism of the collapse of lung units with low inspired ventilation–perfusion ratios ($\dot{V}_{AI}/\dot{Q}$) when high oxygen mixtures are inhaled. *(A)* The expired ventilation is very small because so much of the inspired gas is taken up by the blood. (*C* and *D*) More gas is removed from the lung unit than is inspired, leading to an unstable condition.

blood flow). The reason why so little gas is exhaled is that so much is taken up by the blood. In *B*, where the inspired ventilation is slightly reduced to 44.0 units (same blood flow as before), there is no expired ventilation because all the gas that is inspired is absorbed by the blood. Such a unit is said to have a "critical" ventilation–perfusion ratio.

In Figure 9.6 *C* and *D*, the inspired ventilation has been further reduced with the result that it is now less than the volume of gas entering the blood. This is an unstable situation. Under these circumstances, either gas is inspired from neighboring units during the expiratory phase of respiration as in *C*, or the unit gradually collapse as in *D*. The latter fate is particularly likely if the unit is poorly ventilated because of intermittent airway closure. This is probably common in the dependent regions of the lung in ARDS because of the greatly reduced FRC. The likelihood of atelectasis increases rapidly as the inspired oxygen concentration approaches 100%.

The development of shunts during oxygen breathing is an additional reason why high concentrations of this gas should be avoided if possible in the treatment of patients with respiratory failure. Also, the shunt that is measured during 100% oxygen breathing (Fig. 2.7) in these patients may substantially overestimate the shunt that is present during air breathing.

Retrolental Fibroplasia

If newborn infants with the infant respiratory distress syndrome are treated with high concentrations of oxygen, they may develop fibrosis behind the lens of the eye, leading to blindness. This has been successfully avoided by keeping the arterial P_{O_2} below 140 mm Hg. Recently, however, the disease has reappeared for reasons that are not clear.

10

Mechanical Ventilation

Mechanical ventilation has become increasingly important in the management of patients with respiratory failure. Once used only as an emergency procedure in resuscitation or as a last resort in the treatment of the critically ill, it is now frequently employed to tide a patient over a respiratory crisis. Mechanical ventilation is a complex and technical subject, and this discussion is limited to the physiologic principles of its use, benefits, and hazards.

Intubation and Tracheostomy

Most ventilators require a port for connection to the lung airway. An exception is the tank type of ventilator (see later text), which is now rarely used. The connection is made by means of an endotracheal or tracheostomy tube. These tubes are provided with an inflatable cuff at the end to give an airtight seal. Endotracheal tubes can be inserted via the nose or mouth.

These tubes have additional functions besides providing a connection for ventilators. They facilitate the removal of secretions by suction catheter, a serious problem in many patients with respiratory failure. Retained secretions are particularly troublesome in patients who are obtunded, who have a suppressed cough reflex, or in whom the secretions are particularly copious or viscid. In addition, a tracheostomy may be necessary to bypass upper airway obstruction caused, for example, by allergic edema or a laryngeal tumor. The tube may also prevent the aspiration of blood or vomitus from the pharynx into the lung.

The decision to intubate and ventilate a patient should not be lightly undertaken because it is a major intervention requiring a substantial investment of personnel and equipment, with many potential hazards. However, patients are frequently intubated too late in the course of respiratory failure. The precise timing depends on such factors as the nature of the underlying disease process, the rapidity of the progress of hypoxemia and hypercapnia, and the age and general condition of the patient.

Several complications are associated with the use of endotracheal and tracheostomy tubes. Ulceration of the larynx or the trachea is sometimes seen. This complication is particularly likely if the inflated cuff exerts undue pressure on the mucosa; furthermore, the subsequent scarring can result in tracheal stenosis. The use of large-volume, low-pressure cuffs has reduced the incidence of this problem. Also, care must be taken with the placement of an endotracheal tube. For example, if the distal end of the tube is inadvertently placed in the right main bronchus, atelectasis of the left lung may ensue.

Types of Ventilators

Constant-Volume Ventilators

These ventilators deliver a preset volume of gas to the patient, usually by means of a motor-driven piston in a cylinder (Fig. 10.1) or a motor-driven bellows. The stroke and frequency of the pump can be adjusted to give the required ventilation. The ratio of inspiratory to expiratory time can be controlled by a

Figure 10.1.   Example of a constant-volume ventilator (schematic). In practice, the stroke volume and frequency can be regulated. During the expiratory phase, as the piston descends, the diaphragm is deflected to the left by the reduced pressure in the cylinder, allowing the patient to exhale through the spirometer.

special switching mechanism. Oxygen can be added to the inspired air as required, and a humidifier is included in the circuit.

Constant-volume ventilators are robust, dependable machines that are suitable for long-term ventilation. They are used extensively in anesthesia. They have the advantage of having a known volume (or nearly so) delivered to the patient despite changes in the elastic properties of the lung or chest wall or increases in airway resistance. A disadvantage is that high pressures can be developed; however, in practice, a safety blow-off valve prevents pressures from reaching dangerous levels. Estimating the patient's ventilation from the stroke volume and frequency of the pump may lead to important errors because of the compressibility of the gas and leaks, and it is better to measure the expired ventilation with a spirometer.

Constant-Pressure Ventilators

These ventilators deliver gas at a preset pressure. They do not require electrical power but instead work off a source of compressed gas having a pressure of at least 50 pounds/square inch.

The principle of such a ventilator (Bird) is shown in Figure 10.2. The device

Figure 10.2. Principle of a constant-pressure ventilator (schematic). In *(A)*, the sliding valve is to the right, and gas enters the pressure chamber and is delivered to the patient. When a preset pressure is reached, the diaphragm moves the valve to the left *(B)*, thus cutting off the gas supply, and the patient exhales. (See text for further details.)

consists essentially of two chambers known as the ambient and pressure chambers separated by a diaphragm and sliding valve. During inspiration, shown in Figure 10.2A, the sliding valve is held to the right by the magnet X, and gas enters the pressure chamber. When the preset pressure is reached, the diaphragm is distorted by the pressure across it and forces the valve to the left, thus cutting off the supply of gas (Fig. 10.2B). The resulting change in pressure activates a valve in the line near the patient (not shown in Fig. 10.2), expiration occurs, and the cycle is repeated.

There are several additions to this basic operation. By adjustment of the position of magnet Y, the sliding valve can be held to the left in the exhalation position until the patient makes a small inspiratory effort. The reduced pressure then moves the diaphragm and valve to the right, thus delivering an inspiration to the patient. In this way the ventilator can assist the breathing of a patient in whom this is depressed. Inspiratory flow rate can be controlled by a needle valve in the line to the gas supply and appropriate mixtures of oxygen and air can be delivered. A nebulizer is included in the circuit. In some models, expiration of the patient can be assisted by negative pressure developed by a Venturi device.

Constant-pressure ventilators are small, relatively inexpensive machines. Their chief disadvantage is that the volume of gas they deliver is altered by changes in the compliance of the lung or chest wall. Also, an increase in airway resistance may decrease the ventilation because there may be insufficient time for equilibration of pressure to occur between the machine and the alveoli. Expired volume should therefore be monitored, and this is difficult with some ventilators. Another disadvantage of some constant pressure ventilators is that the inspired oxygen concentration varies with the inspiratory flow rate. Constant-pressure ventilators are now mainly used for "pressure-assist ventilation," i.e., to assist intubated patients overcome the increased work of breathing occasioned by the relatively narrow endotracheal tube. This mode is valuable in weaning patients from a ventilator.

Tank Ventilators

The ventilators we have discussed up to this point are called positive-pressure ventilators because they expand the lung by delivering positive pressure to the airway. By contrast, tank respirators deliver negative pressure (less than atmospheric) to the outside of the chest and rest of the body, excluding the head (Fig. 10.3). They consist of a rigid box ("iron lung") connected to a large volume, low pressure pump that controls the respiratory cycle. The box is often hinged along the middle so that it can be opened to allow nursing care.

Tank ventilators are no longer used in the treatment of acute respiratory failure because they limit access to the patient and because they are bulky and inconvenient. They were employed extensively to ventilate patients with bulbar poliomyelitis and they are still occasionally useful for patients with chronic neuromuscular disease who need to be ventilated for months or years. A modification of the tank ventilator is the cuirass which fits over the thorax and abdomen and also generates negative pressure. It usually is reserved for patients who have partially recovered from neuromuscular respiratory failure.

-10 to zero
cm water

Airtight
seal

To low
pressure pump

Figure 10.3. Tank respirator (schematic). The rigid box is connected to a large volume, low pressure pump which swings the pressure from about 0 to −10 cm H_2O.

Patient-Cycled Ventilators

In these ventilators, the inspiratory phase can be triggered by the patient as he or she makes an inspiratory effort. The term "assisted ventilation" is sometimes given to this mode of operation. An example is the Bird ventilator of Figure 10.2, and generally the constant-pressure machines have this capability. These ventilators are sometimes useful in the treatment of patients who are recovering from respiratory failure and who are being weaned from a period of controlled ventilation.

Patterns of Ventilation

Intermittent Positive Pressure Ventilation (IPPV)

This is sometimes called intermittent positive pressure breathing (IPPB) and is the common pattern in which the lung is expanded by the application of positive pressure to the airway and allowed to deflate passively to FRC. With modern ventilators, the main variables that can be controlled include the tidal volume, respiratory frequency, duration of inspiration versus expiration, the inspiratory flow rate, and the inspired oxygen concentration.

In patients with airway obstruction, there is an advantage in prolonging the expiratory time so that regions of the lung with long time constants have time to empty. (See West JB. Respiratory physiology–the essentials, ed. 5. Baltimore: Williams & Wilkins, 1995: p. 161.) This can be done by reducing the respiratory frequency and increasing the expiratory versus inspiratory time. On the other hand, a prolonged positive airway pressure may impede venous return to the thorax (see later text). Generally, a relatively low frequency and an expiratory time greater than inspiratory time are selected, but each patient requires individual attention.

Positive End-Expiratory Pressure (PEEP)

In patients who have ARDS, considerable improvement in the arterial Po_2 can often be obtained by maintaining a small positive airway pressure at the end of expiration. Values as low as 5 cm H_2O are often beneficial, but pressures as high as 20 cm H_2O or more are sometimes used. Special valves are available to provide the pressure. A secondary gain from PEEP is that it may allow the inspired oxygen concentration to be decreased, thus lessening the risk of oxygen toxicity.

Several mechanisms are probably responsible for the increase in arterial Po_2 resulting from PEEP. The positive pressure increases the FRC, which is typically small in these patients because of the increased elastic recoil of the lung. The low lung volume causes airway closure and intermittent ventilation (or none at all) of some areas, especially in the dependent regions (Fig. 3.5), and absorption atelectasis ensues (Fig. 9.5). PEEP tends to reverse these changes. Patients with edema in their airways also benefit, probably because the fluid is moved into small peripheral airways or alveoli, allowing some regions of the lung to be reventilated.

Figure 10.4 shows the effects of PEEP in a patient with ARDS (46). Note that the level of PEEP was progressively increased from 0 to 16 cm H_2O and

Figure 10.4. Reduction of shunt and increase of dead space caused by increasing levels of PEEP in a patient with adult respiratory distress syndrome (ARDS). Note that as the PEEP was progressively increased from 0 to 16 cm H_2O, the shunt decreased from 43.8 to 14.2% of the cardiac output, and the dead space increased from 36.3 to 49.8% of the tidal volume. (From Dantzker DR, Brook CJ, DeHart P, et al. Ventilation-perfusion distributions in the adult respiratory distress syndrome. Am Rev Respir Dis 1979;120:1039–1052.)

this caused the shunt to fall from 43.8 to 14.2% of the cardiac output. A small amount of blood flow to poorly ventilated alveoli remained. The increase in PEEP also caused the dead space to increase from 36.3 to 49.8% of the tidal volume. This can be explained partly by compression of the capillaries by the increased alveolar pressure and also the increase in volume of the lung and consequent increased radial traction on the airways, which increases their volume. This situation is discussed further on page 163.

Occasionally, the addition of too much PEEP reduces rather than increases the arterial Po_2. Possible mechanisms include: 1) a substantial fall in cardiac output, which reduces the Po_2 of mixed venous blood and therefore the arterial Po_2; 2) reduced ventilation of well-perfused regions (because of increasing dead space and ventilation to poorly perfused regions); and 3) diversion of blood flow away from ventilated to unventilated regions by the raised airway pressure. This deleterious effect of PEEP on the arterial Po_2 is fortunately seldom seen.

PEEP tends to reduce cardiac output by impeding venous return to the thorax, especially if the circulating blood volume has been depleted by hemorrhage or shock. Accordingly, its value should not be gauged by its effect on the arterial Po_2 alone but in terms of the total amount of oxygen delivered to the tissues. The product of the arterial oxygen concentration and the cardiac output is a useful index because changes in this alter the Po_2 of mixed venous blood and therefore the Po_2 of many tissues. Some physicians use the level of the Po_2 in mixed venous blood as a guide to the optimal level of PEEP.

However, in some extremely ill patients, the Po_2 of mixed venous blood can be misleading. Under some conditions, the application of PEEP causes a reduction in overall oxygen consumption of the patient (47). Although this raises the oxygen concentration and Po_2 of mixed venous blood (see equation on page 147), this is not beneficial to the patient. Apparently, the oxygen consumption falls because the perfusion of some tissues is so marginal that if their blood flow is further decreased, they are unable to take up oxygen and presumably slowly die.

Continuous Positive Airway Pressure (CPAP)

Some patients who are being weaned from a ventilator breathe spontaneously but are still intubated. Such patients may benefit from a small positive pressure applied continuously to the airway by a valve system on the ventilator. The improvement in oxygenation results from the same mechanisms as for PEEP. A form of CPAP had been used successfully in the treatment of infant respiratory distress syndrome (IRDS). Another form of CPAP is useful in treating sleep disordered breathing caused by upper airway obstruction.

Intermittent Mandatory Ventilation (IMV)

This is a modification of IPPV (see previous text) in which a large tidal volume is given at relatively infrequent intervals to an intubated patient who is breathing spontaneously. It is often combined with PEEP or CPAP. This pattern may be useful in weaning a patient from a ventilator, and in preventing upper airway occlusion in obstructive sleep apnea by using nasal CPAP during the night.

High Frequency Ventilation

It is possible to maintain normal blood gases by very high frequency (approximately 20 cycles/sec) positive-pressure ventilation with low stroke volumes (50–100 ml). The lung is vibrated rather than expanded in the conventional way, and the transport of the gas occurs by a combination of diffusion and convection. The main use is in patients in whom gas leaks from the lung via a bronchopleural fistula.

Physiologic Effects of Mechanical Ventilation

Reduction of Arterial Pco$_2$

In general, mechanical ventilation is used to increase ventilation and improve pulmonary gas exchange in lungs in which it is grossly defective. This defect may result either because the patient is not able to breathe spontaneously, as in neuromuscular disease, or because the lung itself is severely diseased, as in ARDS. Frequently, mechanical ventilation is begun because the arterial Pco$_2$ is rising or already elevated, and it is usually effective at keeping this in check or reducing it. In patients with airway obstruction in whom the oxygen cost of breathing is high, mechanical ventilation may appreciably reduce the oxygen uptake and CO$_2$ output, thus contributing to the fall in arterial Pco$_2$.

The relationship between the arterial Pco$_2$ and the alveolar ventilation in normal lungs is given by the familiar equation:

$$P_{CO_2} = \frac{\dot{V}_{CO_2}}{\dot{V}_A} \cdot K$$

where K is a constant. In diseased lungs, the denominator $\dot{V}_A$ in this equation is less than the ventilation going to the alveoli because of alveolar dead space, that is, unperfused alveoli or those with high ventilation-perfusion ratios. For this reason, the denominator is sometimes referred to as the "effective alveolar ventilation."

Mechanical ventilation frequently increases both the alveolar and anatomic dead spaces. As a consequence, the effective alveolar ventilation is not increased as much as the total ventilation. This is particularly likely if high pressures are applied to the airway. This can be seen in the example shown in Figure 10.4. As the level of PEEP was increased from 0 to 16 cm H$_2$O in this patient with ARDS, the dead space increased from 36.3 to 49.8%. In some patients, high levels of PEEP also result in the appearance of lung units with high ventilation-perfusion ratios that cause a shoulder to form on the right of the ventilation distribution curve. This did not occur in the example shown. Occasionally, a large physiologic dead space is seen with IPPV even in the absence of PEEP. An example is shown in Figure 8.3.

There are several reasons why positive-pressure ventilation increases dead space. First, lung volume is usually raised, especially when PEEP is added, and the resulting radial traction on the airways increases the anatomic dead space. Next, the raised airway pressure tends to divert blood flow away from ventilated regions, thus causing areas of high ventilation-perfusion ratio or even unperfused areas (Fig. 10.4). This is particularly likely to happen in the uppermost regions of the lung where the pulmonary artery pressure is relatively low because of the hydrostatic effect. (See West JB. Respiratory physiology–the essentials, ed. 5, Baltimore: Williams & Wilkins, 1995: p. 41.) Indeed, if the pressure in the capillaries falls below airway pressure, the capillaries may collapse completely, resulting in unperfused lung (Fig. 10.5) (48). This collapse is encouraged by two factors: 1) the abnormally high airway pressure, and 2) the reduced venous return and consequent hypoperfusion of the lung. The latter is particularly likely to occur if there is a reduced circulating blood volume (see later text).

The tendency for the arterial Pco_2 to rise as a result of the increased dead space can be countered by resetting the ventilator to increase the total ventilation. Nevertheless, it is important to remember than an increase in mean airway pressure can cause a substantial rise in dead space, although the increased pressure may be necessary to combat the shunt and resulting hypoxemia (Fig. 10.4).

In practice, many patients who are mechanically ventilated develop an abnormally low arterial Pco_2 because they are overventilated. This results in a respiratory alkalosis that frequently coexists with a metabolic acidosis because of the hypoxemia and impaired peripheral circulation. An unduly low arterial Pco_2 should be avoided because it reduces cerebral blood flow and therefore contributes to cerebral hypoxia.

Another hazard of overventilation in patients with CO_2 retention is a low serum potassium, which predisposes to abnormal heart rhythms. When CO_2 is retained, potassium moves out of the cells into the plasma and is excreted by the kidney. If the Pco_2 is then rapidly reduced, the potassium moves back into the cells, thus depleting the plasma.

Increase in Arterial Po_2

In some patients with respiratory failure, for example, those with ARDS, the arterial Pco_2 is typically not raised and the objective of mechanical ventilation is to increase the Po_2. In practice, such patients are always ventilated with oxygen-enriched mixtures, and the combination is often effective in relieving the hypoxemia. The inspired oxygen concentration should ideally be sufficient to raise the arterial Po_2 to at least 60 mm Hg, but unduly high inspired concentrations should be avoided because of the hazards of oxygen toxicity and atelectasis.

In some patients with severe forms of ARDS, intermittent positive pressure ventilation with 100% O_2 is not successful in raising the arterial Po_2 to 60 mm Hg. In these circumstances, the life-threatening hypoxemia of these patients can often be relieved by the addition of PEEP of 5–20 cm H_2O (Fig. 10.4). As noted earlier, this probably acts in several ways. The resulting increase in lung volume opens up atelectatic areas and reduces intermittent airway closure, particularly in the dependent regions. Also, edema fluid in the larger airways is moved peripherally, thus allowing some previously obstructed areas to be ventilated.

Figure 10.5. Effect of raised airway pressure on the histological appearance of pulmonary capillaries. *(A)* Normal appearance. *(B)* Collapse of capillaries when alveolar pressure is raised above capillary pressure. (From Glazier JB, Hughes JMB, Maloney JE, et al. Measurements of capillary dimensions and blood volume in rapidly frozen lungs. J Appl Physiol 1969;26:65–76.)

Figure 10.6. Effect of mechanical ventilation on venous return. The diagram shows typical pressures at the end of inspiration. A, atmospheric pressure; V, peripheral venous pressure (mm Hg). The pressure across the chest wall is indicated by the *downward arrow*; this is zero (except for spontaneous respiration), because at this lung volume the chest wall is in its relaxed position. Transpulmonary pressure is represented by the *upward arrow*. Note that the pressure gradient responsible for venous return is reduced by IPPV and tank respirators but not by the cuirass type. (From Sykes M K, McNicol MW, Campbell EJM. Respiratory failure, 2nd ed. Oxford: Blackwell, 1976.)

As an example, the patient whose lung biopsy is shown in Figure 8.2 was put on 10 cm H_2O PEEP on the day after the biopsy was taken. This resulted in a rise in arterial Po_2 of 80 to 130 mm Hg during 80% oxygen breathing.

Effects on Venous Return

Mechanical ventilation tends to impede the return of blood into the thorax and thus reduce the cardiac output. This is true both for positive-pressure and negative-pressure ventilation. In a supine, relaxed patient, the return of blood to the thorax depends on the difference between the peripheral venous pressure and the mean intrathoracic pressure. If the airway pressure is increased by a ventilator, mean intrathoracic pressure rises and venous return is impeded (Fig. 10.6) (49). Even if airway pressure remains atmospheric, as in a tank respirator (Fig. 10.3), venous return tends to fall because the peripheral venous pressure is reduced by the negative pressure. Only in the cuirass respirator is venous return virtually unaffected.

The effects of positive-pressure ventilation on venous return depend on the magnitude and duration of the inspiratory pressure and, particularly, the addition of PEEP. The ideal pattern from this standpoint is a short inspiratory phase of relatively low pressure followed by a long expiratory phase and zero (or slightly negative) end-expiratory pressure. However, such a pattern encourages a low lung volume and consequent hypoxemia, and a compromise is generally necessary.

An important determinant of venous return is the magnitude of the circulating blood volume. If this is reduced, for example, by hemorrhage or shock, positive-pressure ventilation often causes a marked fall in cardiac output. Systemic hypotension may ensue. It is therefore important to correct any volume depletion by appropriate fluid replacement. The central venous pressure is often monitored as a guide to this but should be interpreted in the light of the increased airway pressure. Positive airway pressure itself raises central venous pressure. An additional factor often contributing to the fall in cardiac output during mechanical ventilation is hypocapnia caused by overventilation.

Miscellaneous Hazards

Mechanical problems are a constant hazard. They include power failure, broken connections, and kinking of tubes. Apnea alarms are available to warn of these dangers, but skilled care by the intensive care team is essential.

Pneumothorax can occur, especially if PEEP and/or unusually large tidal volumes are used. Interstitial emphysema may develop if the lung is overdistended. The air escapes from ruptured alveoli, tracks along the perivascular and peribronchial interstitium (Fig. 6.1), and may enter the mediastinum and the subcutaneous tissue of the neck.

Pulmonary infection is a danger if the equipment is not scrupulously clean. Crusting of the large airways occurs unless the gas is efficiently humidified. Cardiac arrhythmias may be caused by rapid swings in pH and hypoxemia. There is also an increased incidence of gastrointestinal bleeding in these patients.

Symbols, Units, and Normal Values

Symbols

Primary

C   Concentration of gas in blood
F   Fractional concentration in dry gas
P   Pressure or partial pressure
Q   Volume of blood
$\dot{Q}$ Volume of blood per unit time
R   Respiratory exchange ratio
S   Saturation of hemoglobin with O_2
V   Volume of gas
$\dot{V}$ Volume of gas per unit time

Secondary Symbols for Gas Phase

A   Alveolar
B   Barometric
D   Dead space
E   Expired
I   Inspired
L   Lung
T   Tidal

Secondary Symbols for Blood Phase

a   arterial
c   capillary
c′   end-capillary
i   ideal
v   venous
$\bar{v}$ mixed venous

Examples

O_2 concentration in arterial blood Ca_{O_2}
Fractional concentration of N_2 in expired gas Fe_{N_2}
Partial pressure of O_2 in mixed venous blood $P\bar{v}_{O_2}$

Units

Traditional metric units have been used in this book. Pressures are given in mm Hg; the torr is an almost identical unit.

In Europe, SI (Système International) units are now commonly used. Most of these are familiar, but the kilopascal, the unit of pressure, is confusing at first. One kilopascal = 7.5 mm Hg.

Conversion of Gas Volumes to BTPS

Lung volumes, including FEV and FVC, are conventionally expressed at body temperature (37°C), ambient pressure, and saturated with water vapor (BTPS). To convert volumes measured in a spirometer at ambient temperature (t), pressure, saturated (ATPS) to BTPS, multiply by

$$\frac{310}{273 + t} \cdot \frac{P_B - P_{H_2O}(t)}{P_B - 47}$$

In practice, tables are available for this conversion (3).

The derivation of this equation and all the other equations is given in the companion volume. (West JB. Respiratory physiology–the essentials, ed. 5. Baltimore: Williams & Wilkins, 1995: pp. 168–172)

Reference Values

Reference Values for Lung Function Tests

Normal values depend on age, sex, height, weight, and ethnic origin. This is a complex subject, and for a detailed discussion the reader is referred to pages 445–513 of Cotes JE. Lung function. 5th ed. Oxford: Blackwell, 1993. Reference values for some commonly used tests are shown in Table A-1. References 50 and 51 contain additional useful discussions of normal values. There is evidence that people are becoming healthier and that lung function is improving.

Table A-1. Example of Reference Values for Some Commonly Used Pulmonary Function Tests in White Non-smoking Adults in the United States

	Men	Women
TLC (l)	7.95 St + 0.003 A − 7.33 (0.79)	5.90 St − 4.54 (0.54)
FVC (l)	7.74 St − 0.021 A - 7.75 (0.51)	4.14 St − 0.023 A − 2.20 (0.44)
RV (l)	2.16 St + 0.021 A − 2.84 (0.37)	1.97 + 0.020 A − 2.42 (0.38)
FRC (l)	4.72 St + 0.009 A − 5.29 (0.72)	3.60 St +0.003 A − 3.18 (0.52)
RV/TLC (%)	0.309 A + 14.1 (4.38)	0.416 A + 14.35 (5.46)
FEV_1 (l)	5.66 St − 0.023 A − 4.91 (0.41)	2.68 St − 0.025 A − 0.38 (0.33)
FEV_1/FVC (%)	110.2 − 13.1 St − 0.15 A (5.58)	124.4 − 21.4 St − 0.15 A (6.75)
FEF_{25-75} (ls^{-1})	5.79 St − 0.036 A − 4.52 (1.08)	3.00 St − 0.031 A − 0.41 (0.85)
$MEF_{50\% FVC}$ (ls^{-1})	6.84 St − 0.037 A − 5.54 (1.29)	3.21 St − 0.024 A − 0.44 (0.98)
$MEF_{25\% FVC}$ (ls^{-1})	3.10 St − 0.023 A − 2.48 (0.69)	1.74 St − 0.025 A − 0.18 (0.66)
DI (ml min^{-1} $mmHg^{-1}$)	16.4 St − 0.229 A + 12.9 (4.84)	16.0 St − 0.111 A + 2.24 (3.95)
DI/V_A	10.09 − 2.24 St − 0.031 A (0.73)	8.33 − 1.81 St − 0.016 A (0.80)

St is stature (height) (m), A is age (years). Standard deviation is in parentheses. From Cotes JE. Lung function. 5th ed. Oxford: Blackwell, 1993.

Appendix B

References

1. Standardization of Spirometry–1987 update. Am Rev Respir Dis 1987;136:1285–1298.
2. Guy HJB, Prisk GK, Elliott AR, et al. Inhomogeneity of pulmonary ventilation during sustained microgravity as determined by single-breath washouts. J Appl Physiol 1994;76:1719–1729.
3. Cotes JE. Lung function. 5th ed. Oxford: Blackwell, 1993.
4. Hinson KFW. Diffuse pulmonary fibrosis. Hum Pathol 1970;1:275–288.
5. Riley RL, Cournand A. "Ideal" alveolar air and the analysis of ventilation-perfusion relationships in the lung. J Appl Physiol 1949;1:825–847.
6. Wagner PD, Laravuso RB, Uhl RR, et al. Continuous distributions of ventilation-perfusion ratios in normal subjects breathing air and 100% O_2. J Clin Invest 1974;54:54–68.
7. Flenley DC. Another non-logarithmic acid-base diagram? Lancet 1971;1:961–965.
8. Bates DV, Macklem PT, Christie RV. Respiratory function in disease. 2nd ed. Philadelphia: WB Saunders, 1971.
9. Nadel JA, Comroe Jr, JH. Acute effects of inhalation of cigarette smoke on airway conductance. J Appl Physiol 1961;16:713–716.
10. Read DJC. A clinical method for assessing the ventilatory response to carbon dioxide. Austral Ann Med 1967;16:20–32.
11. Whitelaw WA, Derenne JP, Milic-Emili J. Occlusion pressure as a measure of respiratory center output in conscious man. Respir Physiol 1975;23:181–199.
12. Lane DJ, Howell JBL. Relationship between sensitivity to carbon dioxide and clinical features in patients with chronic airways obstruction. Thorax 1970;25:150–159.
13. Jones NL. Exercise testing in pulmonary evaluation. N Engl J Med 1975;293:541–544, 647–650.
14. Jones NL, Campbell EJM, Edwards RHT, et al. Clinical exercise testing. Philadelphia: WB Saunders, 1975.
15. Heard BE. Pathology of chronic bronchitis and emphysema. London: Churchill, 1969.
16. Lucey EC, Stone PJ, Snider GL. Consequences of proteolytic injury. In: Crystal RG, West JB, Weibel ER, Barnes PJ, eds. The lung: scientific foundations, 2nd ed. New York: Raven Press, 1997.
17. Thurlbeck WM. Chronic airflow obstruction in lung disease. Philadelphia: WB Saunders, 1976.
18. Burrows B, Fletcher CM, Heard BE, et al. The emphysematous and bronchial types of chronic airways obstruction. Lancet 1966;1:830–835.
19. Colebatch HJH, Finucane KE, Smith MM. Pulmonary conductance and elastic recoil relationships in asthma and emphysema. J Appl Physiol 1973;34:143–153.
20. Wagner PD, Dantzker DR, Dueck R, et al. Ventilation-perfusion inequality in chronic pulmonary disease. J Clin Invest 1977;59:203–206.
21. Macklem PT. Airway obstruction and collateral ventilation. Physiol Rev 1971;51:368–436.

171

22. Cherniack RM, Cherniack L, Naimark A. Respiration in health and disease, 2nd ed. Philadelphia: WB Saunders, 1972.
23. Weiss EB, Segal MS, Stein M. Bronchial asthma. Mechanisms and therapeutics. 2nd ed. Boston: Little, Brown, 1985.
24. Barnes P, Rodger I, Thompson N. Asthma: basic mechanisms and clinical management. New York: Academic Press, 1988.
25. Weibel ER. Morphological basis of alveolar-capillary gas exchange. Physiol Rev 1973;53:419–495.
26. Weibel ER, Gil J. Structure-function relationships at the alveolar level. In: West JB, ed. Bioengineering aspects of the lung. New York: Marcel Dekker, 1977.
27. Gracey DR, Divertie MB, Brown AL Jr, et al. Alveolar-capillary membrane in idiopathic interstitial pulmonary fibrosis. Electron microscopic study of 14 cases. Am Rev Respir Dis 1968;98:16–21.
28. Hamman L, Rich AR. Acute diffuse interstitial fibrosis of the lungs. Bull Johns Hopkins Hosp 1944;74:177–212.
29. West JB. Ventilation-perfusion relationships. Am Rev Respir Dis 1977;116:919–943.
30. Treatment of sarcoidosis. Am Rev Respir Dis 1971;103:433–434.
31. Crone C, Saumon G, Basset G. News from the alveoli. NIPS 1990;5:50–53.
32. Staub NC. The pathophysiology of pulmonary edema. Hum Pathol 1970;1:419–432.
33. West JB, Mathieu-Costello O. Vulnerability of pulmonary capillaries in heart disease. Circulation 1995;92:622–631.
34. Severinghaus JW, Swenson EW, Finley TN, et al. Unilateral hypoventilation produced in dogs by occluding one pulmonary artery. J Appl Physiol 1961;16:53–60.
35. Dantzker DR, Wagner PD, Tornabene VW, et al. Gas exchange after pulmonary thromboembolization in dogs. Circ Res 1978;42:92–103.
36. D'Alonzo GE, Bower JS, DeHart P, et al. The mechanisms of abnormal gas exchange in acute massive pulmonary embolism. Am Rev Respir Dis 1983;128:170–172.
37. Gonda I. Particle deposition in the human respiratory tract. In: Crystal RG, West JB, Weibel ER, Barnes PJ, eds. The lung: scientific foundations. 2nd ed. New York: Raven Press, 1997.
38. Heppleston AG, Leopold JG. Chronic pulmonary emphysema: anatomy and pathogenesis. Am J Med 1961;31:279–291.
39. Ulmer WT, Reichel G. Functional impairment in coal worker's pneumoconiosis. Ann NY Acad Sci 1972;200:405–412.
40. Bone RC, George RB, Hudson LD. Acute respiratory failure. New York: Churchill Livingstone, 1987.
41. Canonico AE, Brigham KL. Biology of acute injury. In: Crystal RG, West JB, Weibel ER, Barnes PJ, eds. The lung: scientific foundations. 2nd ed. New York: Raven Press, 1997.
42. Lamy M, Fallat RJ, Koeniger E, et al. Pathologic features and mechanisms of hypoxemia in adult respiratory distress syndrome. Am Rev Resp Dis 1976;114:267–284.
43. Farrell PM, Avery ME. Hyaline membrane disease. Am Rev Respir Dis 1975; 111:657–688.
44. West JB, Wagner PD. Pulmonary gas exchange. In: West JB, ed. Bioengineering aspects of the lung. New York: Marcel Dekker, 1977.
45. Kapanci U, Weibel ER, Kaplan HP, et al. Pathogenesis and reversibility of the pulmonary lesions of oxygen toxicity in monkeys. Lab Invest 1969;20:101–118.
46. Dantzker DR, Brook CJ, DeHart P, et al. Ventilation-perfusion distributions in the adult respiratory distress syndrome. Am Rev Respir Dis 1979;120:1039–1052.
47. Danek SJ, Lynch JP, Weg JG, et al. The dependence of the oxygen uptake on oxygen delivery in the adult respiratory distress syndrome. Am Rev Respir Dis 1980; 122:387–395.
48. Glazier JB, Hughes JMB, Maloney JE, et al. Measurements of capillary dimensions and blood volume in rapidly frozen lungs. J Appl Physiol 1969;26:65–76.

49. Sykes MK, McNicol MW, Campbell EJM. Respiratory failure. 2nd ed. Oxford: Blackwell, 1976.
50. Clausen JL, ed. Pulmonary function testing guidelines and controversies. New York: Academic Press, 1982.
51. American Thoracic Society. Lung function testing: selection of reference values and interpretative strategies. Am Rev Resp Dis 1991;144:1202–1218.

Appendix C

Further Reading

The list of references (page 171) provides additional information about some specific topics referred to in the text. Other sources of general interest are as follows.

Lung Function Tests and What They Mean

Cherniack RM, Cherniack L. Respiration in health and disease. 3rd ed. Philadelphia: WB Saunders, 1983.
Cotes JE. Lung function. 5th ed. Oxford: Blackwell, 1993.
Fishman AP. Assessment of pulmonary function. New York: McGraw Hill, 1980.
Murray JF. The normal lung. 2nd ed. Philadelphia: WB Saunders, 1986.
Nunn JF. Applied respiratory physiology. 4th ed. Oxford: Butterworths, 1993.
West JB. Ventilation/bloodflow and gas exchange. 5th ed. Oxford: Blackwell, 1990.
Wilson AF. Pulmonary function testing: indications and interpretations. Orlando: Grune & Stratton, 1985.

Function of the Diseased Lung

Most of the books listed above. In addition:

Brewis RAL, Gibson GJ, Geddes DM. Respiratory medicine. 2nd ed. London: Ballière Tindall, 1995.
Crystal RG, West JB, Weibel ER, Barnes PJ, eds. The lung: scientific foundations. 2nd ed. New York: Raven Press, 1997.
Fauci AS, ed. Harrison's principles of internal medicine. 14th ed. New York: McGraw Hill, 1998.
Flenley DC. Respiratory medicine. 2nd ed. London: Ballière Tindall, 1990.
Hasleton PS, ed. Spencer's pathology of the lung. 5th ed. New York: McGraw-Hill, 1996.
Murray JF, Nadel JA. Textbook of respiratory medicine. 2nd ed. Philadelphia: WB Saunders, 1994.
Seaton A, Seaton D, Leitch AG. Crofton and Douglas's respiratory diseases. 4th ed. Oxford: Blackwell, 1989.
Thurlbeck WM, Churg AM, eds. Pathology of the lung. 2nd ed. New York: Thieme, 1995.

Function of the Failing Lung

Appropriate sections of the books listed above. In addition:

Bone RC, George RB, Hudson LD. Acute respiratory failure. New York: Churchill Livingstone, 1987.
Scanlon CL. Egan's fundamentals of respiratory care. 6th ed. St. Louis: CV Mosby, 1995.

Appendix D

Questions

(For answers see page 185)
Note: when several possible answers are given, more than one may be correct.

Chapter I

1. Define (a) 1 sec forced expiratory volume, and (b) forced expiratory flow.
2. Maximum flow rate during most of a forced expiration is normally limited by: (a) turbulence in the trachea, (b) rate of contraction of the respiratory muscles, (c) action of the diaphragm, (d) compression of the airways, (e) abdominal muscles.
3. During most of a forced expiration, what pressure difference is responsible for the flow rate?
4. Which of the following factors may reduce the FEV_1 in a patient with COPD? (a) excessive secretions in the airways, (b) reduction in number of small airways, (c) loss of radial traction on airways, (d) loss of elastic recoil of lung, (e) respiratory acidosis.
5. Which of the following factors may contribute to an abnormally high forced expiratory flow rate (in relation to lung volume) in a patient with advanced interstitial fibrosis? (a) hypertrophy of abdominal muscles, (b) increased lung elastic recoil, (c) increased radial traction on the airways.
6. Which of the following results suggest an increased resistance of the peripheral small airways? (a) reduced peak flow rate, (b) low maximal flow rate at 10% VC, (c) reduced vital capacity.
7. The inspiratory flow–volume curve is particularly valuable for (a) measuring the response to bronchodilator drugs, (b) differentiating between chronic bronchitis and emphysema, (c) detecting fixed upper airway obstruction.
8. In a patient with lung disease who has a reduced $FEF_{25-75\%}$, a plot of maximum expiratory flow rate against static elastic recoil pressure shows a normal relationship. This suggests: (a) reduced elastic recoil but normal airways, (b) obstructed airways and reduced elastic recoil, (c) normal elastic recoil but diseased airways.
9. In a patient with mild lung disease, which of the following factors are likely to be responsible for an increased slope of phase 3 (alveolar plateau) in the single breath N_2 test? (a) uneven time constants within the lung, (b) series inequality of ventilation, (c) airway closure in the dependent regions, (d) cardiogenic oscillations.
10. The closing volume as determined from a single breath N_2 test: (a) is most informative in patients with severe pulmonary disease, (b) is thought to reflect the state of small peripheral airways, (c) is highly reproducible in normal subjects, (d) normally increases with age.
11. After an upright normal subject takes a vital capacity breath of pure O_2, the N_2 concentration at the apex exceeds that at the base because: (a) airway closure at the base delays filling of that region, (b) airway resistance of lower zones is high, (c) the ventilation–perfusion ratio is high at the apex, (d) the apical alveoli expand less than those at the base.

Chapter 2

1. The oxygen electrode: (a) is a sensitive pH meter, (b) measures the EMF (voltage) developed by the O_2 in a sample of blood, (c) measures the current flowing through a buffer of given Po_2, (d) consumes O_2.
2. In peripheral capillaries, more O_2 can be unloaded from blood at a given Po_2 when: (a) blood temperature is reduced, (b) Po_2 is raised, (c) blood pH is raised, (d) concentration of 2, 3-DPG in the red cells is raised.
3. A young man with normal lungs takes an overdose of barbiturate and hypoventilates. Which of the following will probably reach the value of 50 first (assume usual units)? (a) arterial Po_2, (b) arterial O_2 saturation, (c) arterial Pco_2, (d) plasma bicarbonate concentration.
4. In a patient who has severe diffuse interstitial fibrosis of the lung, factors that are likely to contribute to the hypoxemia on exercise include: (a) reduced alveolar ventilation, (b) reduced time spent by the blood in the pulmonary capillaries, (c) ventilation-perfusion inequality.
5. What is meant by the term ideal alveolar Po_2?
6. What technique can be used to determine the distribution of ventilation-perfusion ratios in the lung of a patient with chronic obstructive pulmonary disease?
7. Why is a patient with $\dot{V}A/\dot{Q}$ inequality able to maintain a normal arterial Pco_2 but not Po_2 by increasing the ventilation to his alveoli?
8. A previously well patient takes an overdose of a narcotic drug and is brought to the emergency room, where the arterial Pco_2 is found to be 80 mm Hg. What value would you expect for the arterial pH?
9. A patient with chronic pulmonary disease undergoes emergency surgery. Postoperatively, the arterial Po_2, Pco_2, and pH are 50, 50 (mm Hg), and 7.20, respectively. What terms would best describe the probable acid-base status?
10. Which of the following factors probably contribute to the reduced diffusing capacity for CO in a patient with emphysema? (a) loss of pulmonary capillaries, (b) reduced elastic recoil, (c) uneven distribution of ventilation, blood flow and diffusion properties, (d) increased FRC.

Chapter 3

1. Which of the following typically results in an increased FRC? (a) emphysema, (b) attack of asthma, (c) pulmonary sarcoidosis, (d) pulmonary embolism, (e) normal aging.
2. In a patient with bullous lung disease, it was found that the FRC as determined in the body plethysmograph was much greater than that measured by helium dilution. Possible explanations include: (a) some regions of the lung were very poorly ventilated, (b) some regions were completely unventilated, (c) some regions had a high blood flow in relation to lung volume.
3. In which of the following conditions is the elastic recoil of the lung typically increased? (a) interstitial fibrosis, (b) attack of asthma, (c) emphysema, (d) mitral stenosis, (e) normal aging.
4. Which of the following factors may contribute to the increase in airway resistance in asthma? (a) edema of airway walls, (b) contraction of bronchial smooth muscle, (c) abnormal secretions in the airway, (d) increased alveolar Pco_2.
5. Which of the following factors may contribute to the impaired ventilatory response to inhaled CO_2 in a patient with COPD? (a) increased inspiratory work for a given ventilation, (b) increased compliance of the chest wall, (c) reduced neural output of the respiratory center, (d) arterial hypoxemia.
6. During an exercise test in a patient with mitral stenosis, it was found that the

respiratory exchange ratio rapidly rose above 1 at a low level of exercise. What were the probable reasons?

7. The apex, compared with the base, of the upright lung has: (a) less blood flow, (b) less ventilation, (c) smaller alveoli, (d) smaller mechanical stresses, (e) less tendency for closure of small airways.

Chapter 4

1. What is meant by the term "emphysema"?
2. What is the typical topographical distribution within the lung of: (a) centriacinar emphysema, (b) emphysema caused by a_1-antitrypsin deficiency, (c) panacinar emphysema.
3. A current hypothesis for the pathogenesis of emphysema is (a) destruction of lung elastin by excessive production of neutrophil elastase, (b) damage to pulmonary capillaries by increased alveolar pressure, (c) chronic stimulation of bronchial mucous glands by cigarette smoking.
4. a_1-antitrypsin deficiency: (a) causes severe bronchitis with emphysema, (b) results in emphysema at a relatively early age, (c) is genetically determined, (d) is common in heterozygotes for the Z gene, (e) particularly affects the apices of the lung.
5. What is the Reid index of chronic bronchitis?
6. Patients with COPD of type A (as opposed to type B) tend to have: (a) more cough productive of sputum, (b) larger lung volumes, (c) lower lung elastic recoil, (d) more hypoxemia, (e) more hypercapnia, (f) lower diffusing capacity, (g) greater tendency to develop cor pulmonale.
7. In a patient who has severe chronic bronchitis and emphysema, which of the following is/are likely to be normal? (a) FEV_1, (b) FVC, (c) FEV_1/FVC, (d) $FEF_{25-75\%}$, (e) $Vmax_{50\%}$, (f) forced expiratory time.
8. If airway conductance (Y) is plotted against static transpulmonary pressure (X), what are the typical findings in patients with: (a) pure emphysema, (b) asthma?
9. What is the chief mechanism of hypoxemia in patients with chronic obstructive pulmonary disease? (a) hypoventilation, (b) diffusion impairment, (c) shunt, (d) ventilation–perfusion inequality?
10. Factors responsible for the increased pulmonary artery pressure in patients with chronic obstructive pulmonary disease include (a) destruction of parts of the pulmonary capillary bed, (b) hypoxic vasoconstriction on low $\dot{V}A/\dot{Q}$ areas, (c) polycythemia (d) smooth muscle hypertrophy in some small arteries, (e) systemic hypoxemia.
11. Abnormal features of the bronchi in asthma include: (a) hypertrophied smooth muscle, (b) hypertrophy of mucous glands, (c) edema of bronchial walls, (d) mucous plugging of some airways, (e) collapse because of destruction of surrounding parenchyma, (f) hypertrophy of cilia.
12. The following play a role in the genesis of the asthma attack: (a) mast cell degranulation, (b) airway inflammation, (c) release of platelet-activating factor (PAF), (d) stimulation of eosinophils, (e) increased cholinergic tone.
13. Mediators responsible for the bronchoconstriction in asthma probably include: (a) histamine, (b) angiotensin, (c) bradykinin, (d) norepinephrine, (e) leukotrienes.
14. Administration of isoproterenol to a patient with asthma frequently reduces the arterial Po_2. The probable reason is: (a) increase in cardiac output, (b) selective bronchodilation in high $\dot{V}A/\dot{Q}$ areas, (c) selective vasodilation in low $\dot{V}A/\dot{Q}$ areas, (d) hypoventilation, (e) decrease in FRC.
15. The diffusing capacity for CO in patients with uncomplicated asthma is typically: (a) low, (b) normal, (c) high.
16. An inhaled foreign body most frequently enters the: (a) left lung, (b) right lung, (c) no preference.

Chapter 5

1. The type 2 epithelial cell (*a*) provides most of the structural support for the normal alveolar wall, (*b*) can multiply and line a damaged alveolar wall, (*c*) can transform into a type 1 epithelial cell, (*d*) secretes surfactant, (*e*) has a very active metabolism.
2. Histologic changes in diffuse interstitial pulmonary fibrosis may include: (*a*) infiltration of the alveolar wall with lymphocytes and plasma cells, (*b*) increase in collagen in the interstitial space, (*c*) possible progression to "honeycomb lung," (*d*) sometimes a cellular exudate within the alveoli, (*e*) increased size of the pulmonary capillary bed.
3. Features of diffuse interstitial pulmonary fibrosis typically include: (*a*) dyspnea, especially on exercise, (*b*) prominent cough productive of copious purulent sputum, (*c*) hemoptysis, (*d*) crepitations in both lungs, (*e*) radiologic changes.
4. Pulmonary function tests in diffuse interstitial pulmonary fibrosis typically show: (*a*) low FEV_1, (*b*) low FVC, (*c*) low $FEV_1/FVC\%$, (*d*) low TLC, (*e*) increased airway resistance (related to lung volume).
5. The hypoxemia of a patient with diffuse interstitial pulmonary fibrosis: (*a*) typically worsens on exercise, (*b*) is chiefly caused by $\dot{V}A/\dot{Q}$ inequality, (*c*) may be partly caused by diffusion impairment, (*d*) is usually associated with CO_2 retention, (*e*) may be worse during exercise than would otherwise be the case because of the abnormally small increase in the cardiac output.
6. Possible factors contributing to the high ventilation during exercise in a patient with diffuse interstitial pulmonary fibrosis include: (*a*) hypoxic stimulation of peripheral chemoreceptors, (*b*) stimulation of intrapulmonary stretch receptors, (*c*) stimulation of central chemoreceptors by an increased arterial Pco_2, (*d*) use of abnormally high tidal volumes.
7. The diffusing capacity for CO in a patient with diffuse interstitial lung disease: (*a*) is typically substantially reduced, (*b*) shows an abnormally small rise during exercise, (*c*) is reduced partly by thickening of the blood gas barrier, (*d*) is reduced partly because of obliteration of pulmonary capillaries, (*e*) falls only very late in the disease.
8. Features of Farmer's lung include: (*a*) hypersensitivity to spores in moldy hay, (*b*) histologic changes primarily in the airways rather than the alveoli, (*c*) restrictive pattern of pulmonary function late in the disease, (*d*) variable amounts of airway obstruction shortly after exposure to the antigen.
9. The following can lead to interstitial pulmonary fibrosis: (*a*) paraquat ingestion, (*b*) oxygen poisoning, (*c*) cigarette smoking, (*d*) radiation to the lung, (*e*) administration of the drug busulfan.
10. Pneumothorax (*a*) may occur spontaneously in apparently fit young adults, (*b*) is usually gradually absorbed in the absence of treatment, (*c*) when present in the tension form is a medical emergency, (*d*) may occur as a complication of mechanical ventilation, (*e*) increases FVC.
11. Pulmonary function tests in severe scoliosis typically show: (*a*) an increased FRC, (*b*) hypoxemia, (*c*) a high work of breathing, (*d*) increased pulmonary artery pressure.

Chapter 6

1. Factors determining the movement of fluid across the walls of pulmonary capillaries include: (*a*) the hydrostatic pressure in the interstitial space, (*b*) the colloid osmotic pressure of the interstitial fluid, (*c*) the permeability of endothelial cells to water and crystalloids, (*d*) the capillary hydrostatic pressure.
2. In the earliest stages of pulmonary edema: (*a*) fluid tracks through the interstitial space to the perivascular and peribronchial spaces, (*b*) there is an increase in lung lymph flow, (*c*) fluid floods alveoli one by one, (*d*) interstitial hydrostatic pressure probably rises, (*e*) cuffs of fluid collect around the small arteries and veins.

3. When edema fluid is present in the airways: (*a*) hypoxemia occurs as a result of shunts, (*b*) the alveoli that contain fluid become overexpanded, (*c*) frothing of the fluid may occur because of the presence of surfactant, (*d*) during positive pressure ventilation the fluid is moved peripherally.

4. Increased permeability of pulmonary capillaries can be caused by: (*a*) inhaled chlorine gas, (*b*) circulating endotoxin, (*c*) oxygen poisoning, (*d*) inflation of the lung to a high volume with PEEP, (*e*) radiation to the lung.

5. High-altitude pulmonary edema (*a*) is probably caused by an increased capillary permeability as a result of the hypoxia, (*b*) is most common in people who acclimatize for long periods, (*c*) is a trivial condition needing no treatment, (*d*) may be related to the high pulmonary artery pressures caused by hypoxic vasoconstriction, (*e*) is best treated by moderate exercise.

6. Severe pulmonary edema with alveolar filling causes: (*a*) reduced lung compliance, (*b*) increased airway resistance, (*c*) hypoxemia that may persist during O_2 breathing, (*d*) rapid shallow respiration.

7. The formation of venous thrombi is favored by: (*a*) dehydration, (*b*) congestive heart failure, (*c*) anemia, (*d*) use of oral contraceptives, (*e*) pregnancy.

8. Presenting features of pulmonary embolism often include: (*a*) pleuritic pain, (*b*) hemoptysis, (*c*) tachycardia, (*d*) pleural friction rub, (*e*) large opacity on the chest radiograph.

9. Moderately large pulmonary emboli often cause: (*a*) arterial hypoxemia, (*b*) increased physiologic dead space, (*c*) some rise in pulmonary artery pressure, (*d*) decreased lung elastic recoil, (*e*) decreased airway resistance.

10. Cor pulmonale: (*a*) may complicate long-standing COPD, (*b*) always results in a reduced cardiac output, (*c*) may occur in advanced restrictive lung disease, (*d*) causes neck vein engorgement, (*e*) causes ankle edema.

Chapter 7

1. Carbon monoxide (*a*) is the most abundant pollutant in urban atmospheres by weight, (*b*) comes chiefly from power stations and industrial plants, (*c*) is a component of cigarette smoke, (*d*) in the concentrations existing on some freeways, can impair mental skills, (*e*) reduces the Po_2 of arterial blood.

2. Inhaled cigarette smoke (*a*) increases the risk of bronchial carcinoma, (*b*) increases the risk of coronary heart disease, (*c*) reduces airway resistance, (*d*) stimulates the autonomic nervous system, (*e*) can raise the blood level of carboxyhemoglobin to 10%.

3. Concerning the deposition of aerosols in the lung: (*a*) many of the largest particles are removed by impaction in the nose and nasopharynx, (*b*) many of the smallest particles ($<$ 1 μm) penetrate to the alveoli, (*c*) many inhaled small particles (0.5 μm) are exhaled on the next expiration, (*d*) the small airways are a favored site for sedimentation, (*e*) deposition is reduced on exercise.

4. In the mucociliary system: (*a*) the mucus comes only from goblet cells lining the bronchial epithelium, (*b*) the cilia beat intermittently about 10 times/min, (*c*) the mucous film normally moves at about 1 mm/min in the trachea, (*d*) the mucous film is probably abnormal in asthma, (*e*) the cilia can be paralyzed by inhaled cigarette smoke.

5. Alveolar macrophages (*a*) engulf foreign particles that deposit in the alveoli, (*b*) can migrate to the mucociliary escalator, (*c*) can be killed by ingested silica, (*d*) may kill ingested bacteria before these are removed from the alveoli, (*e*) secrete alveolar surfactant.

6. Simple coal miner's pneumoconiosis (*a*) is a direct result of inhaling large amounts of coal dust, (*b*) may progress to "progressive massive fibrosis," (*c*) typically causes striking cough and dyspnea at rest, (*d*) causes a fine mottling on the chest radiograph, (*e*) causes a marked reduction in the diffusing capacity for CO.

7. With regard to asbestos-related disease: (a) this may occur in men employed in pipe-lagging, (b) it can cause diffuse interstitial fibrosis, (c) it is associated with an increased incidence of bronchial carcinoma, (d) mesothelioma may occur long after light exposure, (e) asbestos fibers in the sputum can often be recognized.

8. Concerning byssinosis: (a) it is caused by exposure to wool fibers, (b) it causes wheezing and dyspnea, (c) pulmonary function tests show a reduced FEV_1, FVC, and $FEV_1/FVC\%$, (d) the symptoms are worst when the patient returns to work after a 2- or 3-day absence, (e) the disease progresses to diffuse interstitial pulmonary fibrosis.

9. Concerning bronchial carcinoma: (a) the disease has a higher prevalence in urban as opposed to rural communities, (b) the disease is more common in males than in females, (c) the specific carcinogenic agent in cigarette smoke is known, (d) pulmonary function tests are important in the early detection of the disease, (e) a carcinoma is always visible on a good chest radiograph.

10. In cystic fibrosis: (a) the disease is confined to the lungs, (b) affected children invariably die before the age of 15, (c) finger clubbing does not occur, (d) analysis of the sweat is useful in screening, (e) uneven ventilation is an early abnormality of pulmonary function, (f) the gene responsible for the disease has been identified.

Chapter 8

1. Severe hypoxemia can cause: (a) tachycardia, (b) lactic acidemia, (c) retinal hemorrhages, (d) mental clouding, (e) proteinuria.

2. CO_2 retention causes: (a) acidosis, (b) reduced cerebral blood flow, (c) renal retention of bicarbonate, (d) mental clouding, (e) raised CSF pressure.

3. A patient was admitted to hospital with an acute pulmonary exacerbation of chronic pulmonary disease. When given 100% O_2, his arterial Pco_2 increased from 50 to 80 mm Hg. Likely causes were: (a) increase in airway resistance, (b) release of hypoxic vasoconstriction in poorly ventilated areas of lung, (c) depression of ventilation, (d) depression of cardiac output, (e) reduced levels of 2,3-DPG in the blood.

4. Acidosis in respiratory failure is likely to be increased by: (a) depression of ventilation, (b) exacerbation of a chest infection, (c) peripheral circulatory failure, (d) renal retention of bicarbonate, (e) administration of morphine.

5. Features of the adult respiratory distress syndrome (ARDS) include: (a) severe hypoxemia, (b) severe CO_2 retention, (c) reduced lung compliance, (d) reduced FRC, (e) large shunt.

6. The following are thought to play a role in the development of ARDS: (a) damage to capillary endothelial cells, (b) neutrophil accumulation in the lung, (c) release of PAF, (d) generation of oxygen radicals.

7. Features of the infant respiratory distress syndrome include: (a) patchy hemorrhagic edema and atelectasis, (b) absence of pulmonary surfactant, (c) severe hypoxemia, (d) large shunt, (e) increased risk in premature infants.

8. An exacerbation of bronchitis in a patient with advanced COPD typically: (a) increases airway resistance, (b) causes worsening of $\dot{V}A/\dot{Q}$ relationships, (c) causes marked leukocytosis and pyrexia, (d) may result in CO_2 retention, (e) is generally well tolerated without specific treatment.

Chapter 9

1. A young man who was previously well was admitted to the emergency room with barbiturate poisoning that caused severe hypoventilation. When he was given 50% O_2 to breathe, there was no change in his arterial Pco_2. Approximately how much

would his arterial P_{O_2} (mm Hg) be expected to rise? (a) 25, (b) 50, (c) 15, (d) 100, (e) 200.

2. When a patient with severe $\dot{V}_A/\dot{Q}$ inequality was given 80% O_2 to breathe, her arterial P_{O_2} rose to only 300 mm Hg. Factors that might have contributed to this unexpectedly low level include: (a) presence of lung units with very low $\dot{V}_A/\dot{Q}$ values, (b) atelectasis of low $\dot{V}_A/\dot{Q}$ units as a result of the high inspired P_{O_2}, (c) relief of hypoxic vasoconstriction in poorly ventilated areas, (d) loss of alveolar surface area resulting in a low diffusing capacity.

3. A patient with congenital heart disease has a right-to-left shunt and an arterial P_{O_2} of 60 mm Hg during air breathing. When he is given 100% O_2, you would expect his arterial P_{O_2} to rise: (a) not at all, (b) less than 10 mm Hg, (c) more than 10 mm Hg, (d) to about 600 mm Hg.

4. A patient with severe CO poisoning was given an exchange transfusion of stored blood. Measurement of his O_2 dissociation curve showed a marked reduction in P_{50}. Likely causative factors were: (a) arterial CO_2 retention, (b) residual CO level in the blood, (c) abnormally low concentration of 2,3-DPG in the transfused red cells, (d) reduced arterial pH, (e) mild pyrexia.

5. Advantages of nasal cannulas for O_2 administration include: (a) they can be worn comfortably for long periods, (b) inspired O_2 concentrations of up to 60% are readily obtained, (c) the inspired O_2 concentration is accurately known, (d) the inspired P_{CO_2} does not rise.

6. O_2 masks based on the Venturi principle are useful because: (a) they give inspired O_2 concentrations of up to 60%, (b) the inspired O_2 concentration is well controlled, (c) the inspired P_{CO_2} is low, (d) the inspired O_2 concentration increases automatically if the ventilation rises.

7. Uses of hyperbaric O_2 include treatment of: (a) ARDS, (b) severe CO poisoning, (c) gas gangrene infections, (d) spontaneous pneumothorax, (e) some malignant tumors by radiotherapy.

8. Intermittent O_2 therapy may be dangerous in the treatment of respiratory failure because: (a) the arterial P_{CO_2} rises rapidly when the O_2 is stopped, (b) the arterial P_{O_2} falls to very low levels when the O_2 is stopped, (c) the pulmonary artery pressure rises to high levels, (d) systemic hypertension may occur.

9. In pulmonary O_2 toxicity, the first histologic changes probably occur in: (a) type 1 epithelial cells, (b) type 2 epithelial cells, (c) interstitium, (d) capillary endothelial cells, (e) alveolar macrophages.

10. Lung units with low $\dot{V}_A/\dot{Q}$ ratios may collapse when high concentrations of O_2 are inhaled for 1 hour because: (a) pulmonary surfactant is inactivated, (b) O_2 toxicity causes intra-alveolar edema, (c) gas is taken up by the blood faster than it enters the unit by ventilation, (d) interstitial edema around the small airways causes airway closure.

Chapter 10

1. A tracheostomy tube (a) facilitates the removal of secretions by suction, (b) provides a port for mechanical ventilation, (c) can be used to bypass a region of upper airway obstruction, (d) increases the anatomic dead space.

2. Constant-volume ventilators typically (a) do not require electrical power, (b) are small, compact, and portable, (c) provide a nearly constant tidal volume even if lung compliance fails, (d) do not allow the respiratory frequency to be changed.

3. In intermittent positive pressure ventilation, a long inspiratory time: (a) tends to reduce the regional inequality of ventilation, (b) tends to diminish venous return to the thorax, (c) tends to reduce FRC, (d) in general should be avoided in favor of an inspiratory-expiratory time ratio of less than 1.

4. In the treatment of ARDS, the addition of 15 cm H_2O of PEEP typically: (a) increases FRC, (b) reduces shunt, (c) increases alveolar edema, (d) increases physiologic dead space, (e) tends to reduce venous return to the thorax.

5. Mechanical ventilation tends to reduce cardiac output: (a) because it reduces pulmonary vascular resistance, (b) because it reduces the pressure difference responsible for returning venous blood to the thorax, (c) especially if the circulating blood volume is abnormally low, (d) with positive pressure ventilators but not with tank respirators, (e) but even if it does, this cannot reduce tissue Po_2.

6. Hazards of mechanical ventilation include: (a) pneumothorax, (b) raised CSF pressure, (c) interstitial emphysema, (d) pulmonary infection, (e) retinal hemorrhage.

Appendix E

Answers

Chapter 1

1. (a) Volume exhaled in 1 second by a forced expiration from full inspiration. (b) Middle half (by volume) of a forced expiration from full inspiration, divided by its duration.
2. d
3. Alveolar minus intrapleural pressure (approximately).
4. a, b, c, d
5. b, c
6. b
7. c
8. a.
9. a, b
10. b, d
11. d

Chapter 2

1. c, d
2. b, d
3. c
4. b, c
5. P_{O_2} which the lung would have if there were no $\dot{V}_A/\dot{Q}$ inequality and the respiratory change ratio remained the same.
6. Multiple inert gas elimination technique.
7. Because of the different shapes of the O_2 and CO_2 dissociation curves.
8. About 7.2
9. Mixed respiratory and metabolic acidosis.
10. a, c

Chapter 3

1. a, b, e
2. a, b
3. a, d
4. a, b, c
5. a, c
6. Increased elimination of CO_2 following the liberation of lactic acid from hypoxic muscles, and excessive hyperventilation caused by stimulation of intra-pulmonary receptors possibly including J receptors.
7. a, b, e

Chapter 4

1. Disease characterized by enlargement of air spaces distal to the terminal bronchioles, with destruction of their walls.
2. (a) Upper zone, (b) lower zone, (c) no preference, or possibly lower zone.
3. a
4. b, c
5. Ratio of thickness of mucous glands to bronchial wall.
6. b, c, f
7. None
8. (a) Almost normal, (b) displaced to right with reduced slope.
9. d
10. a, b, c, d
11. a, b, c, d
12. All
13. a, c, e

14. *c*
15. *b* or *c*
16. *b*

Chapter 5

1. *b, c, d, e*
2. *a, b, c, d*
3. *a, d, e*
4. *a, b, d*
5. *a, b, c, e*
6. *a, b*
7. *a, b, c, d*
8. *a, c, d*
9. *a, b, d, e*
10. *a, b, c, d*
11. *b, c, d*

Chapter 6

1. *a, b, d*
2. *a, b, d, e*
3. *a, c, d*
4. All
5. *d*
6. *a, b, c, d*
7. *a, b, d, e*
8. *a, b, c, d*
9. *a, b, c*
10. *a, c, d, e*

Chapter 7

1. *a, c, d*
2. *a, b, d, e*
3. *a, b, c, d*
4. *d, e*
5. *a, b, c, d*

6. *a, b, d*
7. All
8. *b, c, d*
9. *a, b*
10. *d, e, f*

Chapter 8

1. All
2. *a, c, d, e*
3. *b, c*
4. *a, b, c, e*
5. *a, c, d, e*
6. All
7. All
8. *a, b, d*

Chapter 9

1. *e*
2. *a, b, c*
3. *c*
4. *b, c*
5. *a, d*
6. *b, c*
7. *b, c, e*
8. *b*
9. *d*
10. *c*

Chapter 10

1. *a, b, c*
2. *c*
3. *a, b, d*
4. *a, b, d, e*
5. *b, c*
6. *a, b, c, d*

Index

Page numbers followed by t and f indicate tables and figures, respectively.